Sugar Addiction No More for Diabetics

A Gut Health Protocol with an Anti-Inflammatory Diet to Detox and Manage Diabetes with Holistic Nutrition (The Blood Sugar Solution for Better Health)

Laura Garrett

Table of Contents

Introduction

My sister and I shared an apartment in our twenties. We both have diabetes and, at the time, pretty serious sugar addictions. Growing up, neither of our parents had diabetes, and our diets consisted mostly of sugar, fat, salt, and more sugar. We frequented fast food joints due to busy schedules and low income. We somehow managed to scrape by on extremely dangerous diets for our conditions, but in doing so, we never truly learned how to eat properly. When we lived together, our behaviors only worsened; we fueled each other's unhealthy eating habits, bringing home pizzas and large sodas and keeping the cabinets stocked with convenience store candy.

One Sunday, I came home from the grocery store to find my sister passed out on the couch. The TV was on, and I assumed that she had fallen asleep as she often did while watching TV. I put away the groceries and then moved to the couch to wake her up. My sister is a pretty heavy sleeper, but I never had any issues waking her up when I needed her to get up. This time, she wouldn't wake up.

I began to panic. I didn't know what could be wrong with her—she was young and had never had any major health complications before, other than her diabetes. I called 911 and rode with her in the ambulance to the hospital. I'm embarrassed to say that when the doctors told me that she had fallen into a diabetic coma, I had never even heard the phrase. I was so vastly uninformed about this health condition that I had been living with for practically all of my life. I realized then that because of this, my sister's life was in danger.

What I thankfully learned shortly after arriving at the hospital was that even though I had been out of the house all morning and afternoon, my sister had likely only fallen into her diabetic coma just before I had returned home. Because of this, she was able to quickly make a full recovery, but I was haunted by all the "what ifs." I was terrified that this would happen again, or that it would happen to me. My sister and

I promised each other that we would start taking our health more seriously, and so, in my mid-twenties, I began to really learn and care about diabetes for the first time.

Having diabetes in combination with a sugar addiction can be extremely dangerous for blood sugar and insulin levels—yet, so many people living with diabetes struggle to curb their sugar addiction. Even if you are aware of the dangers of consuming high levels of sugar as someone with diabetes, changing your behavior is much easier said than done. A sugar addiction and improper diet can also cause a number of other stomach and health issues due to a gut imbalance you may not have even been aware of in the first place. Inflammatory issues are yet another common symptom that you may be experiencing due to all the sugars and toxins you carry in your body. So how do you begin to make a change?

In this book, you will learn how to gradually overcome your sugar addiction and other unhealthy eating habits that may be negatively affecting your blood sugar and insulin levels. You will also learn gut health protocol, allowing you to maintain the gut's natural balance and finally start feeling your best. Through holistic nutrition, you will learn how to incorporate an anti-inflammatory diet that will help you vanquish inflammation, dangerous toxins, and excessive sugars that may be lingering in your body.

This book is designed to help you manage all these symptoms in the long term. It is not filled with trendy fads or impossible-to-maintain diets. I have been where you are today, so I understand the frustration of finding something that works for a brief period but that ultimately leads once again to failure. I spent so many years trying to find a solution to my problem, only to be disappointed in the various methods I tried and myself. I was absolutely disheartened and ready to give up until I started trying the solutions outlined in this book. I've accumulated knowledge on how to make successful and lasting changes in holistic health as someone with diabetes. If I could change my life, I know that you can too.

In fact, you've already taken the first step in deciding to make a change to improve your health and happiness. So with that said, are you ready to begin your journey toward improved diabetic management and overall health?

Part 1:
Sugar Addiction in Gut Health and Diabetes

Chapter 1:

The Diabetes Plague

The body of a person with diabetes produces heightened levels of blood sugar because of irregular production or responses to insulin. Common symptoms of diabetes include frequent urination and increased thirst, unintentional fluctuations in weight, nerve damage that affect sensorial touch, and blood vessel damage which can result in health complications such as vision loss, stroke, heart attack, and kidney disease.

Diabetes is a hormonal and metabolic disease where the body's levels of insulin are deficient and levels of glucose are in excess. As a result, the body cannot metabolize the high amounts of glucose within the body, nor can it properly process amino and fatty acids. When the body cannot properly process glucose, it has to convert the excessive glucose to other substances like glycoproteins and sorbitol. This process can lead to a number of common complications for people with diabetes, such as kidney failure due to heightened labels of protein being processed in the kidneys (Brutsaert, 2022).

The History of Diabetes

Treatment for diabetes is believed to have been first utilized as early as 1550 BC in Egypt. The usage of the word was actually first recorded at around 1425, but the term is believed to have been used as early as 250 BC by Apollonius of Memphis. The full term for diabetes is actually diabetes mellitus, which roughly translates to "pass through sweet" and refers to the heightened levels of glucose within the bloodstream and within the urine of those with diabetes (Porter, 2012).

"Mellitus" was added to the term diabetes in 1675 by Thomas Willis, who was also a major pioneer in the treatment of diabetes, along with Sushruta and Arataeus. Early treatment methods included exercise, wine consumption, overeating (to make up for the fluid weight being lost due to excessive urination), as well as sometimes starvation. Unfortunately, during ancient and medieval times, having diabetes was more often than not a death sentence. However, the known correlation between the disease and sweet urine was vital; in ancient India, people tested for diabetes by placing their urine outside and monitoring it to see if ants flocked to it. If this was the case, they would know that their urine had heightened levels of sugar (Mandal, 2009).

The important correlation between diabetes and the pancreas was discovered in 1889 by Joseph von Mering and Oskar Minkowski, who found that when a dog had its pancreas removed, it would develop diabetes shortly before dying (Mandal, 2009).

The discovery of insulin's role in diabetes was only made in 1910. Sir Edward Albert Sharpey-Schafer discovered that when a person's insulin levels are lacking, they develop diabetes (Mandal, 2009).

Altering one's diet in treatment for diabetes became popularized in 1919, when Dr. Frederick Allen published a book that outlined starvation methods and intense restrictions on the intake of certain foods as a way to manage diabetic symptoms (Mandal, 2009).

A major breakthrough was made in the study of insulin on diabetic patients in 1921 when Charles Herbert Best and Sir Frederick Grant Banting studied the work of Minkowski and Von Mering (who found that removing the pancreas of a dog will lead to diabetes). Best and Banting wanted to reverse this process, and they experimented on dogs who had had their pancreases removed to do so. With these dogs, they transplanted pieces of healthy pancreases into their bodies. Along with a third colleague, Collip, who was able to purify the insulin within the healthy pancreases used for the transplants, they found that in transplanting the new pancreases, the diabetic symptoms of the dogs improved (Porter, 2012).

Because of this, treatment involving insulin became available for people with diabetes beginning in 1922. That same year, a 14-year-old boy named Leonard Thompson became the first diabetes patient to get insulin as a form of diabetes treatment. The boy went on to live for another 13 years, until he passed away from pneumonia. This marked an incredibly significant development in the treatment of diabetes, as it became less of a death sentence, and increasingly treatable (Mandal, 2009).

In 1936, the distinction between type 1 and type 2 diabetes emerged. Sir Harold Percival Himsworth published his findings that outlined the differences between the two types for further study of diabetes as two separate diseases. Himsworth wanted to study why insulin treatment was highly effective for some diabetes patients, while ineffective for other diabetes patients. He found that diabetes patients could be categorized as either insulin-sensitive or insulin-insensitive. We recognize these two groupings today as type 1 and type 2 diabetes (Mandal, 2009).

Throughout the 1960s, diabetes treatment continued to make strides. Urine strips were invented, which provided people with a much more practical and quick way to test for diabetes and also to manage blood sugar levels. The single-use syringe was also invented during this time, which made it much simpler for people to receive insulin injections. In 1969, the portable glucose meter was invented, which gave people a way of monitoring their blood sugar levels on the go. Glucose meters have gotten more and more portable over the years, and today, they are about the size of an iPhone (Porter, 2012).

Insulin pumps were invented in 1970, allowing people to have a steady intake of insulin throughout their day. Today, these pumps are very small and are barely noticeable when worn (Porter, 2012).

Biosynthetic human insulin was first created in 1982. This form of insulin perfectly mirrored natural human-produced insulin and became widely available to diabetes patients during this time (Mandal, 2009).

Until about twenty years ago, type 2 diabetes was not recognized in children. Actually, before this, type 2 diabetes was called "adult-onset diabetes." As doctors noticed more and more children developing the symptoms of type 2 diabetes, however, it was realized that children too could develop this type of diabetes, and thus, the name was changed from "adult-onset" to "type 2." Unfortunately, more and more children continue to receive type 2 diabetes diagnoses because of the rise of mass-produced foods with poor nutrition (such as fast food), childhood obesity, and a lack of exercise (Porter, 2012).

Unfortunately, even through all of the medical and technological advances that have been made in the study and treatment of diabetes, it remains a leading cause of serious health complications and even death worldwide. In fact, according to a 2015 study by the CDC, diabetes was named the seventh most common cause of death in the US (Porter, 2012).

Diabetes and the Black Death: What's the Correlation?

Emerging research has linked the Black Death to certain diseases, including diabetes. Waghorn (2022) provides a detailed explanation of the correlation between the Black Death and diabetes. The Black Death, just like other pandemics, influenced the way in which people's bodies respond to pathogens. However, the Black Death remains the deadliest pandemic in human history, which is why it had such a significant impact on genetic changes in the population. In response to the pandemic, people's genes changed in ways that actually made them increasingly susceptible to autoimmune diseases.

In terms of natural selection, the people who survived the Black Death went on to pass along certain genetic mutations that would protect from such diseases to their offspring. A study using DNA samples in London and Denmark from the teeth of those who died around the time of the Black Death found that Black Death survivors possessed a gene called ERAP2, which would have made them anywhere from 40-50 percent more likely to survive the plague.

However, this gene does not positively impact people's immune systems in the long term. In fact, certain variants of these types of protective genes actually lead to increased risk for autoimmune diseases. During the Black Death, this payoff did not matter nearly as much, as surviving the plague was much more of an urgent matter. Thus, after the Black Death passed, we were left with genes that negatively impacted our autoimmune systems.

Autoimmune disease hinders your body's ability to differentiate between foreign cells and its own cells. As a result, the body ends up fighting its own cells, which it mistakes for foreign cells.

Pandemics typically occur in waves, and in the case of the Black Death, the initial wave was what wiped out the largest number of people. However, as the waves continued over the centuries, fewer and fewer people died from the pandemic because of the prevalence of the ERAP2 gene within a much larger portion of the population.

Food: A Curse and a Cure

"Let food be thy medicine and medicine be thy food." –Hippocrates

We are living in a unique time in history when we have all the necessary knowledge and resources to maintain healthy diets that allow us to live longer and protect us against diseases. However, an overwhelming amount of dangerously unhealthy foods are readily available to the general population. These foods do exactly the opposite of promoting longevity and disease prevention.

In today's world, the quality of our food is getting worse and worse with the influx of foods like doughnuts, french fries, cheeseburgers, candy, and soda, but also with the availability of these kinds of foods. Food delivery apps and fast food joints are taking over the food industry, and as a result, making it easier to dismiss any thought behind choosing what kind of meal you want. People are spending less time in the kitchen focused on creating meals and more time focused on other things, making food less of a priority and more like a second thought.

This type of mindset is invading popular culture, and people who are growing up with this as the norm are the most susceptible to developing dangerous eating habits and diseases such as diabetes from taking in excessive amounts of sugar, fat, and salt. Once they do develop health issues due to their unhealthy diets, they are put on medications to manage their symptoms, and often do not actually change their eating habits. However, the much simpler and holistic solution would be changing their eating habits. Because of this, it is so important to recognize that what we put into our bodies can either nourish or destroy us.

During Hippocrates' time, people recognized the differences between food and medicine. However, food and medicine were not completely separate. Instead, certain foods were often prescribed by doctors to help supplement medicinal treatments. This is because people during this time recognized the correlation between food and overall well-being—something that is often overlooked in today's society, as many people often tend to turn to medicine so they can eat "whatever they want." A prominent example of this is pills or supplements that advertise rapid weight loss while allowing the consumer to eat whatever they want. This type of statement is not only false, but also dangerous because it promotes the idea that there are "miracle cures" to food-related health issues such as obesity. In reality, the only way to truly make a change in your food-related health issue is by changing the types of food you consume. Doing so is much simpler than we often think, but Hippocratic doctors were correct in their belief that food and medicine were inherently linked, and both contributed to holistic well-being (King, 2020).

The Different Types

The most common types of diabetes that we hear about are types one and two. However, many more types of diabetes have been discovered over the years. The four most common types of diabetes are type 1, type 2, prediabetes, and gestational diabetes.

Type 1 diabetes is a type of autoimmune disease, wherein your body is actually attacking its own cells. Specifically, your body does not recognize the cells within your pancreas that produce insulin, and works to destroy them. This type of diabetes can be diagnosed at any age, but it is more commonly diagnosed at younger ages (this is why it used to be called juvenile diabetes, whereas type 2 diabetes was referred to as adult-onset diabetes). If you have this type of diabetes, you will need to take insulin on a daily basis, either by single-use injections or through an insulin pump (Behring, 2021).

With type 2 diabetes (the most common type of diabetes today), your body does not attack its insulin-producing cells. Rather, it simply does not produce enough insulin or does not respond properly to the insulin being produced. Typically, type 2 diabetes is diagnosed in people who are either middle-aged or older. In fact, about 95% of the population with diabetes has this type of diabetes (Behring, 2021).

Prediabetes is the state your body enters just before developing type 2 diabetes. This state is characterized by high levels of blood sugar, but not yet high enough to fall into the category of type 2 diabetes. When left untreated, prediabetes will eventually turn into type 2 diabetes. It's quite common for people to get diagnosed with type 2 diabetes without even realizing that they were prediabetic. This is because diabetic symptoms may be less noticeable in a prediabetic state, which is why it is so important to test blood sugar levels if you know you have a higher risk of developing diabetes (Diabetes UK, 2022).

The good news is, prediabetes is reversible if you catch it in time to take proper action. Regular exercise and a healthy diet (and weight loss resulting from a combination of the two) is the best course of action in reversing prediabetes. When you are able to maintain these healthier lifestyle changes, you can prevent yourself from developing type 2 diabetes.

Behring (2021) provides a detailed account of the following types of diabetes. Gestational diabetes is a type of diabetes that develops while women are pregnant. The good news is, most of the time symptoms go away once the woman is no longer pregnant. But gestational diabetes is an indicator that you have a heightened risk of developing type 2 diabetes. If you have or had gestational diabetes, it is extremely important to practice regular exercise and maintain a healthy diet in order to prevent the development of type 2 diabetes. It is also crucial to test blood sugar levels so that you are able to recognize if you do develop type 2 diabetes.

Another classification of diabetes, called type 4 diabetes, is currently being studied. This type of diabetes is not linked to autoimmune conditions, nor is it linked to weight. Instead, type 4 diabetes seems to be related to age. Insulin resistance has been observed in older people who are not overweight or obese. It is believed that since it is in the earlier research stages, this type of diabetes affects many people who have not been diagnosed. Without weight as a risk for the development of diabetes, and without a clear known cause, it is much harder to determine whether an individual is at risk for this type of diabetes.

In a 2015 study, researchers found that type four diabetes may likely have to do with a higher-than-normal number of T cells (a type of immune cell) combined with the aging process. It is important to spread awareness of this emerging type of diabetes, as it is less likely to be diagnosed at a regular doctor's check-up. Some symptoms to look out for (that are actually quite similar to symptoms of other diabetic types) include: fatigue, frequent urination, increased thirst and hunger, vision issues, unintentional weight fluctuations, and wounds that take longer than normal to heal.

Other types of diabetes that are less common include: monogenic diabetes syndromes, drug or chemical-induced diabetes, cystic fibrosis-related diabetes, and type 3 diabetes, which is another emerging type of diabetes that is still in early research stages.

Who Is at Risk?

The Center for Disease Control and Prevention (2022) provides a detailed account of risk factors for diabetes. Risk factors for type 1 diabetes most commonly include genetics. If you have a known family history of type 1 diabetes, you are more likely to develop it as well. However, other risk factors, as well as steps to take toward risk management, are not currently known. If you know you are at a higher risk for developing this type of diabetes, it is best to regularly check for diabetes as well as stay on the lookout for symptoms indicating that you may have diabetes, such as increased thirst and urination, and unintentional weight loss.

Health issues that affect your pancreas can also lead to the development of type 1 diabetes. Some conditions that damage your pancreas include pancreatic cancer, chronic or acute pancreatitis, pancreatic cysts, bile duct cysts or bile duct cancer, and pancreatic neuroendocrine tumors. These types of conditions can take a toll on your pancreas' ability to produce insulin, which can then lead to type 1 diabetes. Additionally, certain infections or illnesses, though usually quite rare, can have a similarly damaging effect on your pancreas.

The risk factors for type 2 diabetes are much more well-known and recognizable. According to the CDC (2022), if you identify with the following, you may be at risk for type 2 diabetes:

- If you currently or have previously had prediabetes

- If you have a family history of type 2 diabetes

- If you are overweight

- If you are about 45 years old or older

- If you are Latino, Black, or Native American

- If you lead a sedentary lifestyle

- If you have previously had gestational diabetes

- If you have liver disease

The best way to prevent and manage type 2 diabetes is through healthy lifestyle changes including weight loss, diet, and regular exercise.

Risk factors for developing prediabetes include:

- Being overweight or obese

- Being around 45 years old or older

- Having a family history of prediabetes or type 2 diabetes

- Leading a sedentary lifestyle

- Having a history of gestational diabetes

- Being Latino, Black, or Native American.

Just as with type 2 diabetes, the best way to combat prediabetes is to make a lifestyle change that includes regular exercise, a healthy diet, and weight loss. Remember that prediabetes is reversible. However, once your prediabetes develops into type 2 diabetes, that is no longer the case. Because of this, it is best to tackle holistic changes to your health and well-being when you are at risk of or are in a prediabetic stage instead of once you have already developed type 2 diabetes.

You have a higher risk of developing gestational diabetes if you:

- Have previously had gestational diabetes during an earlier pregnancy

- Are overweight or obese

- Have previously given birth to a baby who weighed over nine pounds

- Are over 25 years old

- Have a family history of prediabetes, type 2 diabetes, or gestational diabetes

- Have polycystic ovary syndrome

- Are Latina, Black, or Native American.

Following a pregnancy with gestational diabetes, it is important to monitor your health and check for symptoms of type 2 diabetes, as well as monitor your child's health and risk factors for developing type 2 diabetes. Children born from a gestational-diabetic pregnancy are more likely to go on to develop type 2 diabetes (and also gestational diabetes if they become pregnant later in life). Prevention methods for gestational diabetes are the same as those for type 2 diabetes: maintaining a healthy diet, regular exercise, and weight loss for those who are overweight or obese.

Being overweight or obese tremendously increases your risk of developing type 2, gestational, or prediabetes (CDC, 2022). It can also be extremely dangerous to remain overweight or obese once developing diabetes or prediabetes. If you are overweight and at risk or already have diabetes, it is important to talk to your doctor about losing weight. Generally speaking, a healthy diet and regular exercise is the best way to go about losing weight. You may also be interested in finding out your body mass index, which you can speak to your doctor about. There are also methods for roughly calculating your body mass index yourself. Finding out your body mass index can help you see more specifics in terms of your body makeup.

Typically, an adult is considered overweight once they hit a body mass index of 25 or higher (NIDDK, 2019). This means that you are already at a higher risk for developing type 2 diabetes, or if you already have type 2 diabetes, you are at a higher risk for complications.

To calculate your body mass index, divide your weight (lbs) by your height squared (inches), and then multiply this number by 703: [lbs ÷ (in squared)] x 703. For example, let's say you weigh 150 lbs and are 5'5" (65 inches). Your calculation would be as follows: [150 ÷ (65 squared)] x 703 = 24.96. This would put you at just under overweight, but you may want to consult your doctor to see if you should try to lose weight. Regardless, keeping up a healthy diet and exercise routine should be a priority.

Calculating your waist circumference is another way to estimate if you are at a higher risk for type 2 diabetes. Generally speaking, men who have a waist circumference of over 40 inches and women who are not pregnant and have a waist circumference of over 35 inches are at a higher risk of developing type 2 diabetes. Calculating waist circumference is a way to roughly estimate how much fat is stored in your abdomen area. Unfortunately, even if you do have a body mass index that falls in the healthy range, you may be at a higher risk of developing type 2 diabetes, as well as heart disease, if you carry most of your fat in your abdomen area (NIDDK, 2019).

The Complications of This Disease

Diabetes UK (2022) provides a detailed account of possible diabetes complications. Complications from diabetes can come in the form of acute, which can spring up at any time, or chronic, which tends to build up more gradually. Complications will commonly arise when blood sugar levels are not properly managed. When a person with diabetes has sustained periods of high blood sugar levels, their blood vessels can become damaged. Once this happens, blood flow becomes restricted, which means that the body's organs are not receiving the oxygen-rich blood they need to properly function. It also limits nerve function, which is actually a common complaint among people with diabetes. If the nerves and blood vessels of a person's body become damaged, serious health complications may arise. For instance, lack of circulation and nerve damage in the feet can cause devastating heart complications.

While high blood sugar is probably the risk factor that you hear the most about, complications can also arise due to smoking, excessive alcohol consumption, excessive fat consumption, and high blood pressure. All of these issues are contributing factors to blood vessel damage.

According to Diabetes UK (2022), some acute complications in patients with diabetes include:

- Hypos: A state in which your body's blood sugar levels are too low.

- Hypers: A state in which your body's blood sugar levels are too high.

- Diabetic ketoacidosis: A serious condition that requires immediate medical attention. The body may enter this state due to high blood sugar levels in combination with a lack of insulin, which can then cause an excess of ketones to build up. Ketones are a type of chemical acid that your liver produces in response to not having enough insulin to turn glucose into energy. When the liver is unable to do this, it will then turn to fat to use for energy. When fat is transferred into energy, it becomes what is known as ketones, which are then sent through your bloodstream for your body to use as its energy source.

- Hyperosmolar hyperglycaemic state: This occurs in people with type 2 diabetes. It is also a serious condition that requires immediate medical attention. People with type 2 diabetes can enter this state if they become severely dehydrated or their blood sugar levels become extremely elevated.

Although these complications are acute, they can eventually lead to chronic complications. Some chronic complications include:

- Gum disease, as well as other issues in the mouth, can be caused by heightened blood sugar levels, as this can add more sugar to your saliva. With excessive glucose in your saliva, bacteria can grow more easily in your mouth, which can lead to higher acidity levels within the mouth that damage your gums and tooth enamel. Your gum's blood vessels may also get damaged, which makes infection more likely.

- Kidney problems can arise from high blood pressure and high blood sugar levels, which make it increasingly difficult for the kidneys to rid your body of excess fluids and waste.

- Nerve damage is a symptom that can be caused by elevated blood sugar levels. Once this happens, your nerves may have trouble sending messages between parts of your body and your brain, which can then cause further difficulties such as vision, hearing, mobility, and sense of touch problems.

- Foot problems, which are extremely serious in diabetic patients, can lead to amputation. Catching any foot-related issues as early as possible is the best way to avoid this. A combination of nerve damage, which may affect your ability to maintain proper feeling in your feet, and heightened blood sugar levels, which may lead to blood vessel damage that affects circulation, can make injuries a lot more difficult to heal. If you notice any kind of changes to your feet, it is crucial that you speak to your doctor as soon as possible.

- Heart attack and stroke are major risk factors when blood sugar levels remain regularly heightened, as this damages the blood vessels, which can then lead to a heart attack or stroke.

- Eye problems—most commonly, diabetic retinopathy–which is a type of eye disease that affects vision. If caught early through an eye screening test, it is treatable and vision loss is preventable.

- Cancer that affects organs and areas related to diabetic-related issues. For instance, people with diabetes are at a greater risk of developing pancreatic cancer. Additionally, certain cancer treatments may cause further complications with your diabetes treatment, making it increasingly difficult to manage blood sugar levels.

- Sexual problems can arise when blood vessels and nerves become damaged, thus restricting the amount of blood that is able to flow to the sexual organs. As a result, some loss of feeling can arise within these areas. With women, high blood sugar levels also put the urinary tract at a greater risk of infection.

Taking steps to prevent diabetes-related complications is the best way to avoid them altogether. In fact, taking these preventative steps can also help you manage your diabetes symptoms, as they offer ways to improve your overall health and well-being. The CDC (2022) provides some strategies for preventing diabetes complications. Here are some ways to target these potential problem areas:

- Take care of your heart by maintaining a healthy diet. Heart-healthy foods include fruits, vegetables, lean protein, and whole grains. Try to eat these foods rather than processed foods, sodas, alcohol, and foods that are high in trans fat. Staying active, along with a proper diet, will help you lose weight, which will help lower blood sugar levels and triglycerides (a type of fat that is stored in your blood cells). Increasing your daily physical activity also allows your body to respond more strongly to insulin. By staying active, you not only reduce your risk for heart disease, but also better manage your diabetes. Stress management also helps your heart; when you have chronic stress, you may see elevated blood pressure as well as potentially unhealthy coping mechanisms such as excessive alcohol consumption or binge eating. Seeing a therapist, practicing meditation or breathing exercises, spending quality time with friends and family, and exercising can all help you better manage your stress levels. Regularly getting an A1C test to make sure that your blood sugar levels are where you want them to be, keeping your blood pressure and cholesterol at lower levels, and avoiding smoking are also important steps that you can take to manage your heart health.

- Take care of your kidneys by making sure to stick to your goals for blood sugar levels, remembering to get regular A1C tests (about twice a year for most people, unless your doctor has told you otherwise), and checking your blood pressure regularly to make sure that it is meeting your goals. You will also want to manage your diet by increasing your fruit and vegetable intake and limiting your sodium intake. Create a target cholesterol range with your doctor and regularly check your cholesterol levels. Remember to take all of your necessary medications, and try to spend some time every day being physically active.

- Take steps to prevent nerve damage. Maintaining your target blood pressure levels, getting regular exercise, losing weight (if you are overweight), maintaining a healthy diet, taking your prescribed medications, avoiding smoking, and limiting or avoiding alcohol are all great ways to protect your nerves.

- Managing your foot health can be tricky since sometimes the issue lies with nerve damage. You may not feel anything wrong with your feet, but that doesn't necessarily mean that there isn't a problem. Checking your feet daily for any damage or irregularities is the best way to identify any issues that may arise as early as possible. Wash your feet every day to ensure that they are clean, and try not to walk around barefoot to keep your feet as clean as possible and also to avoid injury (making sure that there is nothing in your shoes, such as a small rock or pebble, before putting them on is also helpful). Only wear shoes that are comfortable and fit well. When you purchase new shoes, it is best to break them in gradually, as opposed to wearing them on a day when you know you'll be walking around a lot. Always wear socks when wearing shoes, and try to opt for closed toe shoes whenever possible. When cutting your toenails, make sure to cut in a straight line, as opposed to curving the edge of the nail in, as this can easily lead to ingrown nails. Use a nail file to ensure there are no sharp edges. If you develop calluses or corns, have a professional work on them instead of trying to get rid of them yourself. Make sure to get your feet checked whenever you go in for a checkup with your doctor, and visit your foot doctor at least once a year. Encourage circulation by putting your feet up or moving your ankles and toes around while sitting down. Engage in activities that promote circulation but that are not too hard on your feet. These kinds of activities can include bicycling, walking, or swimming.

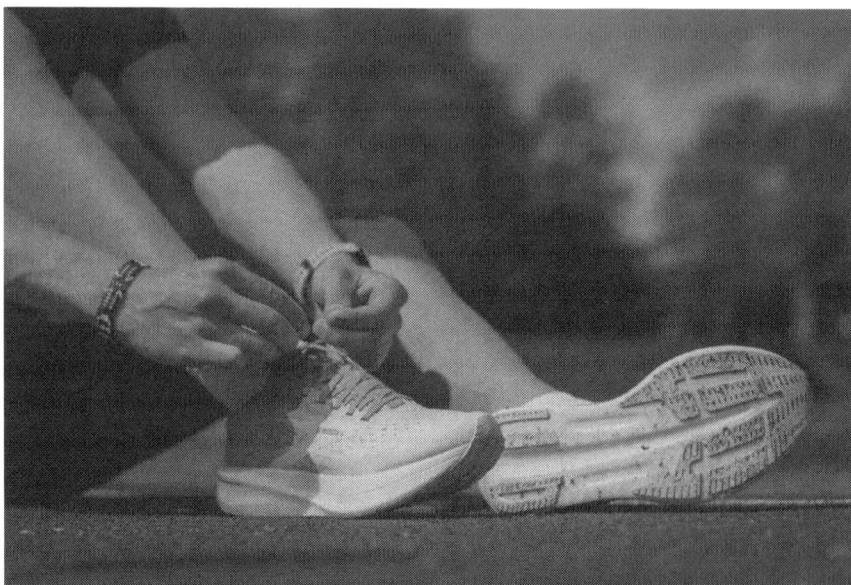

- Maintain optimal oral health. Remember to brush your teeth at least twice per day and floss at least once per day. Make sure that your dentist is aware of your diabetes, and visit your dentist regularly (usually about twice a year, unless otherwise advised). Avoid smoking, as this will put you at higher risk for gum disease as well as cancer, and it can make certain diabetes symptoms worse. If you notice any changes in your oral health, such as irritated gums, visit your dentist to check for gum disease. Make sure to keep track of any symptoms that are bothering you so that you can relay them to your dentist.

- Protect your ears. Maintain yearly hearing tests. Avoid damaging activities such as listening to excessively loud music. Maintain your target range for blood sugar levels. Check with your doctor if any current medication you are on has hearing-related side effects and if there are alternative medications that you can take.

- Take measures to prevent eye disease. Get yearly dilated eye exams to check for and catch eye issues early. Maintain your target blood sugar levels, as elevated blood sugar levels can damage the tiny blood vessels within your eyes over time, as well as alter the shape of your lenses, which will affect your vision. Maintain your target blood pressure and cholesterol levels as well. Avoid smoking, and remember to stay active on a daily basis.

- Take care of your mental health. We often tend to overlook this area when taking steps to improve our diabetes-related health. However, mental health can actually have a huge effect on our physical health. Many people with diabetes have a lot of stress related to their condition. To ease some of this stress, make sure that you have an endocrinologist that you like, as this type of doctor will likely have a more comprehensive understanding and care plan for your diabetes-related worries. It is also beneficial to find a therapist who specializes in chronic health conditions like diabetes. You can also ask your doctor for a referral for this. Finding a diabetes educator can also help you increase your network of people to reach out to when you have questions about your diabetes. Don't try to do everything at once; this can cause more stress than benefits. Instead, it can be more helpful to focus on a few smaller goals at a time, and celebrate each tiny win to motivate you to keep going. Joining a diabetes support group is another helpful option. These groups allow you to speak freely among people who can relate to you and your struggles with diabetes.

Common Myths

Though quite a common chronic disease, there are a lot of myths and misinformation surrounding the topic of diabetes. These myths can be potentially dangerous for those with diabetes, as misinformation can get confused with factual knowledge needed to manage one's symptoms. Tim Newman (2020) provides a detailed account of some common myths related to diabetes. Here are some common myths surrounding diabetes, where they potentially came from, and the truth about these topics:

- Myth: If you don't have a family history of diabetes, you cannot develop diabetes.

    ○ While having a family history of diabetes typically puts you at a greater risk for developing diabetes, anyone can be affected by diabetes. In fact, lots of people with diabetes do not have any immediate family members with diabetes. If you have other risk factors, such as being overweight or having a pancreas condition, you will be at a higher risk for developing diabetes, regardless of whether or not other people in your family have diabetes.

- Myth: All overweight people will eventually develop diabetes.

    ○ While being overweight certainly is a major risk factor for developing type 2 diabetes, being overweight does not necessarily mean that you will develop diabetes. Lots of people who are overweight never develop diabetes, and lots of people who are not overweight do end up developing diabetes. However, this does not put you in the clear either if you are overweight. The best thing to do to help prevent type 2 diabetes if you are overweight is to lose weight through diet and exercise.

- Myth: Only overweight people are at risk of developing diabetes.

    ○ Being overweight is a risk factor for type 2 diabetes, but plenty of non-overweight people also develop diabetes, including type 2.

- Myth: Everyone who eats a lot of sugar will eventually develop diabetes.

- Cutting down on sugar intake is highly encouraged (whether you have diabetes or not). However, sugar itself does not actually cause diabetes. People who do not have diabetes but do consume excess amounts of sugar in their daily diet are more likely to become overweight, which increases their risk of developing diabetes. Because of this, there is a correlation between sugar intake and developing diabetes, but it is not sugar directly that causes a person to develop diabetes.

- Myth: All people with diabetes need to follow the same, restrictive diet.

  - First of all, everyone has different dietary needs, and a diet that works great for one person may not work at all for another person (even if both people have diabetes). Furthermore, being diabetic does not mean that you necessarily need to follow a strict diet; rather, you eat what non-diabetic people eat, but should pay attention to how the foods that you consume affect your blood sugar levels and other areas of concern. Generally speaking, people with diabetes should try to limit foods that are high in sugar, fat, and sodium. However, this is recommended for everyone else as well.

- Myth: People with diabetes can never eat sweets or carbs.

  - People with diabetes should try to limit their sugar intake, but this doesn't mean that they can never consume sugar (this would be realistically impossible). Planning for sugar intake is the best way to go about consuming sugar. Try to limit sweets for special occasions, such as an occasional reward or a celebration. Eating smaller portions of sweets is also recommended when you do eat sweets. Make sure to have a plan, insulin-wise, when you know you will be consuming sweets so that your body is prepared for it. Carbs are also not off-limits for people with diabetes. It is typically recommended to consume carbs in moderation so as not to shock your system. Consuming large amounts of carbs all at once may trigger a sudden change in blood sugar, so eating roughly the same amount of carbs per meal is one way to prevent this from happening. Rather than sources of unhealthy carbs, such as refined carbs and highly processed foods, it is best to get your carb intake from healthy foods such as legumes, whole grains, vegetables, and fruits.

- Myth: Being put on insulin means that you are not managing your blood sugar levels well.

  ○ Needing to take insulin is a regular part of being diabetic. If you have type 1 diabetes, you will need to take insulin because your body does not produce the insulin you need on its own. This does not mean that you are doing something wrong. If you have type 2 diabetes, your body will make less and less insulin over time. Even if you are doing everything right, you will likely need to take insulin in order to manage your blood sugar.

- Myth: You should not exercise if you have diabetes.

  ○ Exercise is a crucial factor in your health, whether you have diabetes or not. In fact, it can actually help manage your diabetes in many ways. Before starting an exercise routine, it is always important to talk to your doctor to make sure that you are choosing an exercise routine that is best for you, as everyone is different and will have different needs and limitations. It is also generally a good idea to start slow; if you have not exercised in a while, start by doing mild to moderate physical activity, such as brisk walking. It's important to build up to more advanced exercises in order to protect your body and see the best results. It's also important to talk to your doctor about any changes in your medications that may be necessary with the addition of exercise in your life. For example, you may need to adjust your insulin dosage around the time you plan to exercise so that your blood sugar levels do not drop too low.

- Myth: If you only have prediabetes, you don't need to worry.

    ○ Prediabetes prevents you from a unique opportunity to actually reverse your condition. It is an indication that if you keep up your unhealthy habits, you will likely develop type 2 diabetes, so you should instead take this time to develop a healthier lifestyle in order to prevent type 2 diabetes. It is important during this time to talk to your doctor to come up with a plan of action. Diet and exercise are essential for reversing prediabetes.

- Myth: Once your blood sugar levels are where you want them to be, you no longer have to take your diabetes medications.

    ○ Taking insulin is necessary for people with type 1 diabetes, and some people with type 2 diabetes are able to manage their diabetes through diet, exercise, and weight loss. However, because diabetes is a progressive disease medication will eventually become necessary, regardless of how healthy a lifestyle you lead. Remember that needing to take medication does not mean that you are doing anything wrong, and it should not be thought of as negative; medication is there to help you manage your blood sugar levels and any other complications that may arise due to your diabetes.

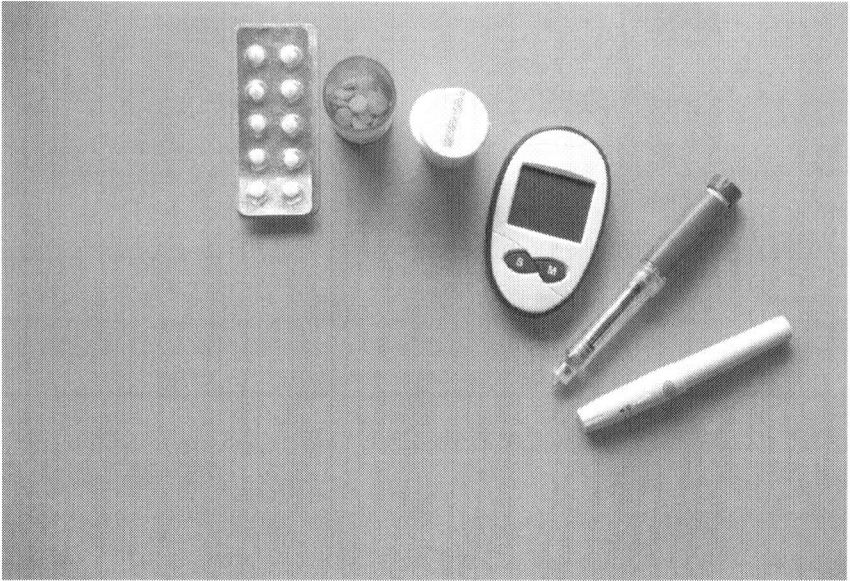

Chapter 2:

Sugar Addiction: The Mountain or the Molehill?

What exactly is sugar addiction? We hear this phrase all the time, but can sugar really be an addictive substance? The short answer is yes. In fact, there is plenty of evidence to suggest that sugar can be addictive in similar ways to substances such as drugs.

Behavioral and neurochemical changes that often occur when people with sugar addictions gain intermittent access to sweets actually mimic those of substance abuse. This kind of intermittent access can over time produce a dependency on the substance (in this case, sugar).

When we consume sugar, our brains release opioids and dopamine, which is what causes it to be actually addictive (Avena et al., 2008). But how addictive is it really? Just as with drugs, sugar makes people want to relive these sensations over and over again, and the only way to chase this high is to consume sugar more frequently and in higher amounts. The more we give into these cravings, the stronger the compulsion grows, which leads the brain to crave more and more as it builds up a tolerance to the substance. As this tolerance builds, we actually need more sugar in order to feel the same "high."

As difficult as it may be to give up sugar, doing so will improve your health in many ways that you may not even expect. Some of these benefits include the obvious ones such as weight loss and more manageable blood sugar levels, but there are also benefits such as better sleep, improved mood, clearer skin, and increased energy throughout the day. When you start to give up sugar, your body will lose some of its built-up tolerance to sugar. This means that when you do have sugar, you will be satisfied with smaller portions and intensity of the sweets you are consuming. It also means that extremely sweet foods that you used to need to achieve a sugar high will likely taste way too sweet (Reichelt, 2017).

When a Sugar High Is Your Quick Fix

There are a lot of reasons why you may feel the overwhelming need to have a sugary snack. For one, sugar is literally addictive, as previously mentioned. The more you develop the habit of consuming sugar, the more difficult it becomes to resist the urge for more. Seidenberg (2018) provides a detailed explanation of some common reasons behind sugar cravings.

Fatigue is also a major cause of sugar cravings. When you feel exhausted, your body craves food that will bring your energy back up. If you are used to this food being sugar, it's what your body will learn to crave. However, foods that are rich in protein and healthy fats will bring your energy up even more successfully because you will not feel that crash once the sugar has quickly worn off. Protein and healthy fats allow your body to use this energy in a more sustained manner, increasing your energy level more steadily. Making sure that you eat healthier foods without skipping meals will help keep your energy up and keep you feeling good without needing to reach for sweets.

Stress is also a huge contributor to sugar cravings. When we are stressed, we naturally want to consume foods that make us feel good. Because sugar triggers a release of serotonin and dopamine in the brain, it can provide us with a quick fix for stress. However, this feeling is extremely brief, and it will not do anything to alleviate stress in the long term. Instead of going for sugar in times of stress, try choosing healthy carbs instead, such as whole grains, legumes, berries, apples, or oranges. These types of foods will produce the same anti-stress response in your brain, as well as nourish your body and make you feel better for much longer than sugar will.

Your gut sends your brain signals when it is craving nutrition. This is your gut's way of telling you that it needs fuel. However, this can easily get misinterpreted as your body craving sugar. Instead of feeding it sugar, nourish your gut with foods like nuts, apples, bananas, or oats, which are high in prebiotic fibers. Doing so will help curb your sugar craving.

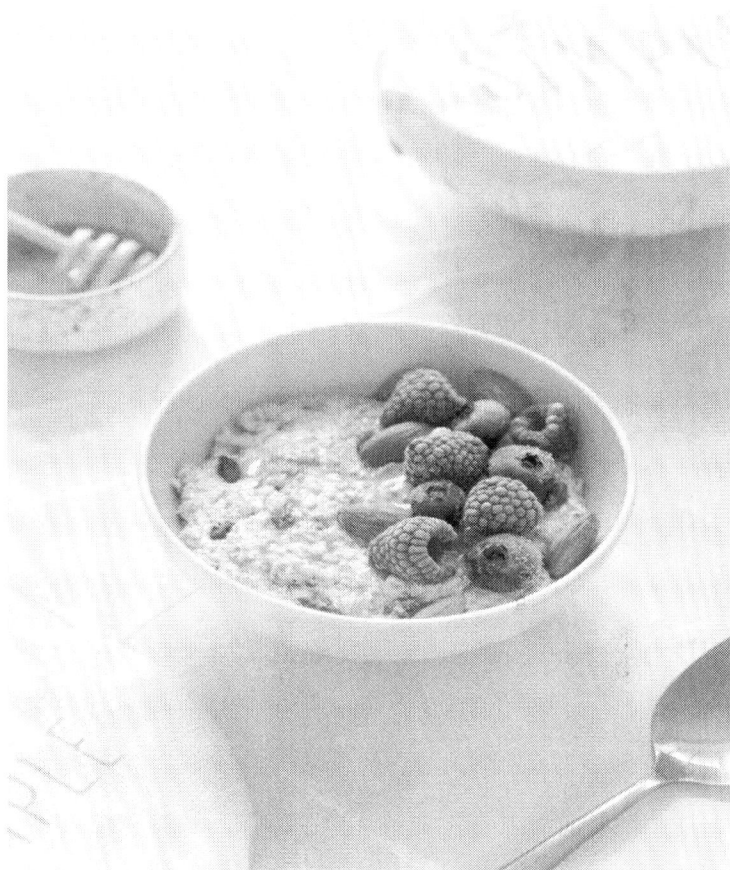

Cut out artificial sweeteners from your diet. They confuse your system because our taste buds can detect sweet flavor, not sugar. Because of this, when people with type 2 diabetes consume artificial sweeteners, the brain signals to the pancreas that it should start producing more insulin to prepare for the "sugar" being consumed, even if what we are consuming is not actually sugar. When this happens, you are at higher risk of hypoglycemia in addition to still craving more sugar or artificial sweetener.

Remember that you are in control over the habits you build! Finding alternative solutions to quick sugar fixes will help you develop healthier habits and start feeling better.

Hormones and Sugar Addiction

Sometimes hormones can cause sugar cravings. Hormonal states such as menstruation, menopause, and andropause can make your body crave carbs and sugar. Hormone deficiencies can also cause these cravings. If you think your cravings might be due to a hormone deficiency, you should talk to your doctor. Other signs of hormone imbalances include fatigue, mood swings, insomnia, decreased sexual libido, weight gain, and high blood pressure. Specifically for females, it is beneficial to pay attention to any other symptoms that may be indicators that your sugar cravings have to do with hormone levels—according to Pelletier (2015), some of these symptoms include:

- a history of pms

- a history of ovarian surgery, or a hysterectomy

- a tendency to have mood swings, depression, anxiety, and bloating a week prior to your period

- a low sex drive

- less than usual vaginal lubrication

- regular hot flashes, insomnia, and headaches

For males, look for symptoms including:

- a low sex drive

- regular erectile dysfunction

- high cholesterol

- high blood pressure

- depression

- being overweight

- type 2 diabetes

That said, it's important to understand that a hormone imbalance may be part of the reason why you have sugar cravings, but sugar can also fuel your hormone imbalance. The Riegel Center (n.d.) provides a detailed account of how hormones can affect sugar cravings. A hormone imbalance leads to an endless cycle of consuming sugar because of the imbalance, only to have the sugar throw your hormones off balance even further. Sugar can actually shut off a gene called SHBG that works to control your sex hormones. Once this occurs, you may start to experience symptoms such as anxiety, fatigue, and mood swings.

The hormone cortisol is triggered in your body when you experience stress. During stress, our fight or flight mode is activated, and in preparation to either fight or flee, our body releases glucose for your muscles to use for energy. This, in turn, makes you crave more sugar.

This is why "stress eating" is such a real and widely-experienced phenomenon. It helps temporarily relieve some of the stress that we are feeling. However, it does nothing to help you in the long term.

Additionally, people with diabetes can actually be affected more significantly by sugar cravings because insulin is one of the hormones that contributes to sugar cravings when deficient. Regulating your insulin and blood sugar levels will help prevent these cravings.

The Role of Anticipation in Sugar Addiction and Reward

Increased sugar consumption, like other addictions, only fuels cravings even further. It alters behavior that mimics behavior associated with addiction. Specifically, it makes us increasingly reward-seeking and increases our anticipation for reward. This is because when we consume sugar, reward molecules like dopamine are released in our bodies. When we form a habit of consuming sugar in order to bring about these sensations, we spend more time thinking about how sugar makes us feel, even when we are not actually eating sugar (Wiss et al., 2018).

The more sugar we eat, the more we reinforce these habits and thought patterns. As a result, we become more impulsive when it comes to sugar consumption. Once this happens, it only becomes harder and harder to resist the urge to eat sugar—and in higher volume. These changes can also trigger other issues like neurological function, which can then have an effect on things like our mood and behavior (Wiss et al., 2018).

When you become addicted to sugar, areas of your brain that also deal with things like anxiety and depression are activated. This can often trigger mental health issues, which can then lead to further reinforcement of addictive behaviors as a coping mechanism (Jaques et al., 2019).

Sugar vs. Substance Addiction

Sugar is often compared to hard drugs when talking about its addictive properties. Dr. William Wilson compares it to cocaine, stating that it has similar effects including "altering mood, possibly through its ability to induce reward and pleasure, leading to the seeking out of sugar" (Davis, 2017, para. 4). However, it is also believed that it is not actually sugar itself that is necessarily addictive, but rather, sweetness. When you consume sweet flavors you want more and over time you develop addictive behaviors around sweet snacks and drinks. However, there doesn't seem to be much difference in effects on human behavior when looking at different types of sugar, including artificial, sugar-free sweeteners.

While there is still ongoing debate within the scientific community regarding sugar and addiction (in particular its comparison to drugs like cocaine), many researchers believe that drugs such as cocaine more severely limit a person's self-control than sugar. Regardless, the comparison—although perhaps not quite as severe as cocaine—is still valid. As Dr. Hisham Ziauddeen outlines, "the brain's rewards system and the circuits that control eating behavior are the same ones that respond to drugs of abuse" (Davis, 2017, para. 13).

How the Standard American Diet Is Ruining Our Health

"[The sugar industry] claimed that there are no bad foods, only bad diets, and these were due to personal choices." –Kaare R. Norum, University of Oslo

Americans consume massive amounts of sugar on a daily basis. In fact, there are often sugars that we are unaware of added to foods we eat. Actually, "more than half of what Americans eat is ultra-processed, and that accounts for 90% of added sugar consumption" (Cumbers, 2021, para. 9). This, in combination with an increasingly sedentary modern American culture, is leading to more and more obesity.

Sugary drinks (and drinks with artificial sweeteners) also sneak sweets into our diet, which spike blood sugar levels (in the case of drinks that use real sugar) and encourage sugar addiction. Sweet beverages are tricky because they are often marketed as healthy. Sports drinks, for instance, are advertised as being especially helpful for hydration and workout recovery. However, what is not being advertised is that they have massive amounts of sugar—often even more sugar in one bottle than we should be consuming in an entire day. These kinds of sneaky sugars that find their way into the typical American diet are why so many people's blood sugar levels are constantly much higher than they should be (Filipovic, 2013).

So many foods and drinks sneak in excessive amounts of sugar because manufacturers know that sugar is addictive. The truth is, companies want us to return time and time again to their product, which is why they use this specific disguised sugar tactic as a way to lure us in and keep us hooked. Because of this, Americans are constantly being fed (both literally and figuratively) a standard diet that makes us sick and even kills us for the purpose of capitalist interest.

Since the food industry is making it more and more difficult every year for Americans to have access to a proper diet, it has become the responsibility of the individual to do everything they can to improve their diet. Unfortunately, this is the most difficult for people in a low-income bracket.

In fact, low-income populations are targeted for unhealthy foods. Low-income neighborhoods often are described as food deserts. This term refers to the way that low-income neighborhoods often do not have any grocery stores nearby where people can purchase healthier foods such as fresh produce. Instead, the food that is sold in their area consists mainly of cheaper, longer-lasting, highly processed foods such as chips, candy, and soda. Because fresh produce is more perishable, stores will often stay away from purchasing fresh produce because it yields greater losses; if people do not purchase their product right away, the store has to take the loss. On the other hand, chips, candy, and soda will not likely make the store take any losses because these types of foods take much longer to expire.

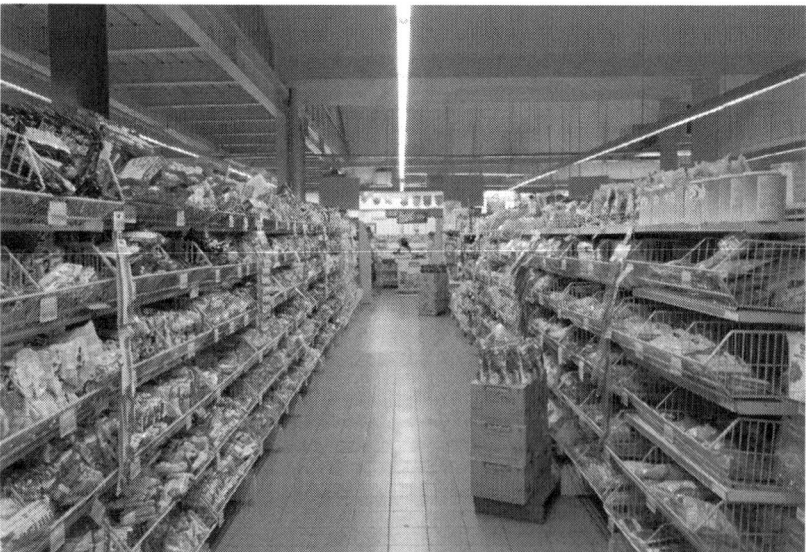

Additionally, because chain restaurants have much more money than small businesses, they are able to spring up almost everywhere, replacing smaller restaurants. These chain restaurants tend to purchase ingredients in bulk, which allows them to produce much larger portions for much less money. As a result, customers eat more food that is scarce in nutritional value. This kind of culture makes it increasingly rare to find fresh, nutritious ingredients in the foods that we eat because we have less and less access to them. This is an issue on a systemic level—and unfortunately, one that we do not yet have a solution for.

Sugar Addiction: Its Role in Obesity and Diabetes

"Americans are having dessert several times a day and don't know it." –Dr. Alan Greene, Institute for Responsible Nutrition

Sugar and sweeteners such as high fructose corn syrup are abundant in the typical American diet. However, the human body is simply not able to process sugar and sweeteners in the quantities that most Americans consume them. Even if you do not eat ice cream and cookies every day, you likely consume much more sugar than you realize. This is because sugars are so well-hidden in so many foods that are advertised as healthy. For instance, having a low-fat yogurt for breakfast may sound like a healthy choice—certainly healthier than opting for chocolate-chip pancakes. But what may not be so obvious is that your low-fat yogurt can have more sugar packed in that little cup than you should be eating in an entire day.

Actually, your daily sugar intake should consist of under 10% of your overall food consumption. It is recommended that less than 100 calories in an adult female's diet should come from sugar. This roughly equates to a maximum of six teaspoons. It is recommended that less than 150 calories in an adult male's diet should come from sugar. This comes out to about nine teaspoons, max. Since one teaspoon equals four grams of sugar, even "a cup of most commercial apple juices— even those labeled 100-percent juice—will max you out for the day" (Krans, 2019, para. 6).

With sweeteners being added to nearly every type of processed food, it's safe to assume that if it's processed, there has been sweetener added and nutrients removed. These sweeteners are dense in calories, which is a major contributor to the rising levels of obesity.

The sugars that are naturally in foods like fruit and dairy are what should be making up your daily sugar intake. When you consume these sugars, you are also consuming nutrients that naturally occur in these foods. On the other hand, foods with added sweeteners only give you sugar without providing any nutritional value. These foods are commonly referred to as "empty calories" for this reason. However, it is more helpful and accurate to actually think of these foods as not being solely "empty" calories, but harmful ones because they harm your body. The word "empty" makes it sound as though these foods neither provide us with any benefits, nor harm us, but in reality they destroy our bodies (Krans, 2019).

Chapter 3:

Shedding Light on the Gut

Microbiome

When we talk about the gut, we are talking about your body's gastrointestinal system. Kho and Lal (2018) provide a detailed account of how your gut health is affected by the bacteria present in its system. Your gut is responsible for digesting your food, and it does so by breaking the food down and then releasing the nutrients through the gut's walls so that they can be carried through your blood. In order to do this, your gut must use a combination of hormones, bacteria, and nerves.

Bacteria helps your gut by forming a layer of mucus along the gut's walls. We tend to think of bacteria as something we need to get rid of, but actually, the health of your gut depends on a balance of good bacteria and bad bacteria.

The bacteria, eukarya, and archaea coexisting in your gut are referred to as gut microbiota. While your gut's main function is digestion, the balance of your gut microbiota also affects many other aspects of the body, including the following:

- mood and mental health

- central nervous system

- immune system

- regulating aches and pains

- strengthening the gut's walls, which protects your body from infectious pathogens

- regulating inflammation

- protecting against serious digestive issues such as crohn's disease, irritable bowel syndrome (ibs), cancers, and ulcerative colitis, having to do with inflammation in the intestines

- metabolism

Microbes in the gut becoming unbalanced can bring about different diseases and conditions. For instance, when unbalanced, the gut's bacteria may not be able to maintain the strengthening mucous lining that protects your gut's walls. As a result, you are at a higher risk of developing infections, digestive conditions like IBS, and autoimmune disorders like celiac disease.

Interestingly, irregularities in the gut microbiota are also associated with obesity. This has to do with the gut's management of the body's metabolism. When the gut microbiota becomes imbalanced, it cannot properly maintain a healthy metabolic rate, so metabolism tends to decline, leading to weight gain. As we know, this is dangerous when it comes to risk factors for type 2 diabetes. Though this area is still being researched, it is believed that taking prebiotics and/or probiotics is a helpful approach to combating this issue.

Gut Health: Does It Affect Everything?

Gut-Brain Connection

In addition to areas like digestion and metabolism, the gut is also linked to other areas of the body. Johns Hopkins Medicine (2019) gives a detailed account of the gut-brain connection. Sometimes referred to as the body's "second brain," the gut plays a role not only in digestion, but also things like your mood and the way you think. This "second brain" is called the enteric nervous system (ENS). The ENS is in constant communication with your brain. It can actually be the trigger for many situations that we often find ourselves in and associate with the brain, such as mood swings. This connection is called the gut-brain axis.

Sometimes the gut's microbiota is thrown off, leading to issues like IBS, aches, and bloating. These gut issues often lead to emotional responses that can actually be quite severe, including depression and anxiety. This is because when the gut is upset, it sends messages to the central nervous system, and because of this, we get these shifts in mood. This is why such a large percentage of people with chronic bowel issues also have anxiety and/or depression.

Since these types of gut and psychological issues are tied, treatment in one area can help in the other area as well. For instance, therapy aimed at treating symptoms of depression can also start to help with bowel issues. In fact, antidepressants can actually help reduce gastrointestinal symptoms, and it is not uncommon for gastroenterologists to prescribe this type of medication to treat a gut issue such as IBS.

The brain and the gut have massive amounts of neurons (the brain has about 100 billion, while the gut has roughly 500 million). The nerves within the body's nervous system connect the neurons of the brain and the gut. One major nerve that is connected in this way is the vagus nerve, which allows your brain and gut to communicate. When we experience stress, our brains may send stress signals through this nerve, and as a result, we may experience gastrointestinal issues. Think about how often your stomach feels upset when you are stressed—this is why! The vagus nerve in people with Crohn's disease or IBS is weakened, thus making effective communication between the brain and the gut more difficult.

Another similarity in the brain-gut axis is with neurotransmitters, which are chemicals that control emotions. These chemicals include neurotransmitters that you have likely heard of, such as serotonin— often labeled the "happy hormone." While you may already know that your brain produces serotonin, you may not be aware that your gut does too.

Another common neurotransmitter that can be seen both in the brain and the gut is gamma-aminobutyric acid (GABA).

This neurotransmitter helps control anxiety and fear. Interestingly, probiotics can help elevate GABA levels, thus reducing symptoms of anxiety (Robertson, 2020).

Gut-Hormone Connection

Dr. Leigh Ann Scott (n.d.) provides a detailed explanation of the gut-hormone connection. The microbiota in the gut is essential in regulating estrogen levels. When it becomes unbalanced, issues related to estrogen imbalance–such as polycystic ovary syndrome, endometriosis, and certain cancers–may arise. This is because when the gut microbiota is unbalanced, it leads to either an excess or deficiency of estrogen levels. When this happens, you can see a wide variety of issues spring up, such as weight gain, which can then contribute to diabetes-related issues.

Imbalance of the gut microbiota can be caused by improper diet and a sedentary lifestyle. Foods containing phytoestrogens can trigger an imbalance in the gut microbiota. But there are ways to counteract these changes.

Probiotics are believed to help balance estrogen levels through balancing the gut microbiota. They work by adding good bacteria to your gut, thus bringing up the count of good bacteria so that the good bacteria in your gut are not overrun by the bad bacteria. This will strengthen your immune system and improve gastrointestinal health.

The gut is also linked to the pituitary gland, which is responsible for making the hormones that help manage your appetite. When the gut becomes unbalanced, it may send out conflicting signals that result in your pituitary gland being confused as to whether you are hungry or full.

Your gut produces a large portion of the serotonin stored in your body. Serotonin, also known as the "happy hormone," is essential in managing your mental health. When your gut is not able to produce enough serotonin, it is common to develop depression and anxiety.

Insulin is also aided by an area in your gut called the *Lactobacillus reuteri*. When the *Lactobacillus reuteri* is affected by inflammation due to an imbalance of gut microbiota, insulin regulation becomes increasingly difficult.

Steps that you can take to improve hormonal symptoms of an unbalanced gut include:

- Adopting an anti-inflammatory diet that is rich in nutrients

- Consuming probiotics and prebiotics

- Steering clear of sugars, artificial sweeteners, trans fats, and processed foods

- Taking antibiotics only when you need to (also taking a probiotic at the same time that you take your antibiotic and doubling down on your probiotic consumption once you are through taking your antibiotics)

- Consuming polyphenols (plant compounds that help digestion and that are naturally occurring in foods like olive oil)

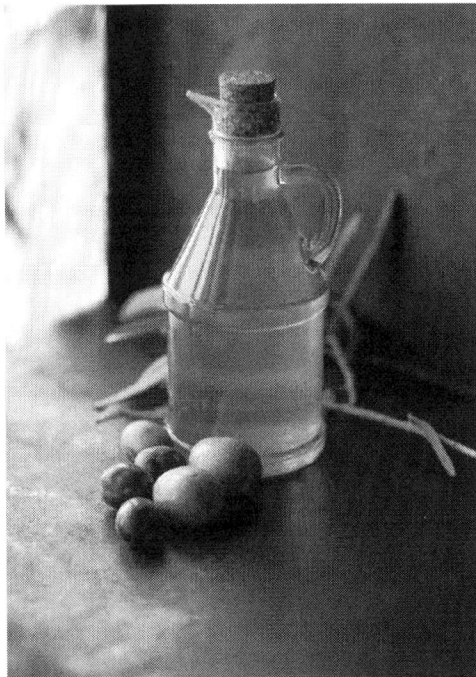

- Increasing your water consumption

Gut-Thyroid Connection

When you have an imbalanced gut microbiota, you are more likely to have an underperforming thyroid. When the thyroid stops working as it should, you have what is called hypothyroidism. Some symptoms of hypothyroidism include hair loss, weight gain, and chronic fatigue.

An unbalanced gut microbiota is extremely common in those with thyroid conditions because gut imbalance promotes inflammation and a declined immune system, which then weakens the gut wall. When this happens, the gut wall cannot guard against the penetration of substances that are meant to stay in the gut. This then leads to increased exposure of the body to inflammation and antigens.

Gut imbalance can also have a direct effect on hormone levels within the thyroid, and the body's mineral absorption rates, which affect how the thyroid functions. When the body cannot absorb minerals like zinc, iron, iodine, and selenium because of a weakened gut, you are likely to end up with thyroid dysfunction. This kind of thyroid dysfunction can then lead to more serious thyroid-related issues–such as thyroid nodules, thyroid cancer, hypo- or hyperthyroidism–if left untreated.

Gut-Sleep Connection

The gut can also affect our quality of sleep. When microbes are depleted within the gut, the gut is no longer able to produce serotonin, which we rely on for healthy sleep cycles. Altering your diet to encourage gut health will help balance your gut microbiota, and as a result, likely help you get better sleep (Huizen 2020).

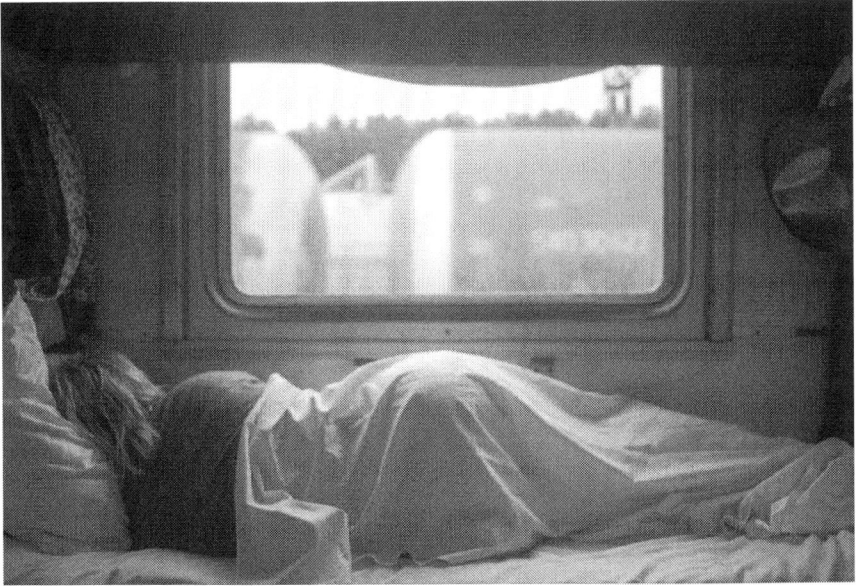

Gut-Food Cravings Connection

The types of food we crave have a lot to do with what is going on in our gut. Interest in this area of research has increased in recent years, and it has been observed that the gut microbes in people with sugar cravings differ from the gut microbes in people who do not crave sugar, even if they consume the exact same diet.

Certain types of bacteria found in the gut produce hormones that manage appetite. The gut will also sometimes produce antibodies that attack these hormones. Because of this, it is believed that microbes can alter food cravings by either producing more or less of these hormones that regulate appetite and also by producing the antibodies that counteract appetite management (Ho, 2014).

Even though we now have this knowledge, more research on the topic still needs to be done to figure out how we can actually take action based on this information. However, the use of prebiotics and probiotics (along with maintaining a healthy, nutritious diet) is known to help manage gut heath, thus allowing us to help balance our gut microbiota.

The Gut's Internal Milieu and Microbiome

Your gut environment is the internal milieu for your microbiome—this is why it is so important to keep your gut as healthy as possible in order to ensure proper conditions for your microbiome to thrive. Your internal milieu is affected by a number of outside factors, including stress, physical environment, medications, age, diet, existing medical conditions, pregnancy, and breastfeeding (Illiano et al., 2020).

Some strategies for regulating your gut environment include probiotic intake, changes to your diet, and lifestyle changes such as increased exercise. Everyone's gut is unique, as your microbiome begins developing at birth and goes through rapid changes during childhood.

As adults, our gut microbiome is still changing and adapting, but typically at slower rates than experienced during childhood. When the gut microbiome changes significantly as an adult, it is usually due to either environmental or genetic factors, or often a combination of the two.

Gut Microbiota and Inflammation: Where They Intersect

A healthy and balanced gut microbiota regulates inflammatory conditions, but when it is unbalanced, it is less capable of protecting against inflammation. In fact, certain microbes, such as unhealthy bacteria known as *Enterobacteriaceae*, can trigger certain inflammatory conditions such as obesity or IBS (Lobionda et al., 2019).

Once this begins to happen, it becomes increasingly difficult for your body to get a handle on inflammatory issues, as the bad bacteria overpopulate and replace the good bacteria. This is where taking steps such as increasing probiotic intake can help restore your good bacteria.

With obesity, the body produces excess cytokines, which leads to chronic inflammation. When diabetic patients have chronic inflammation due to obesity, they are especially at risk of developing complications. This is because this kind of chronic inflammation can actually further promote insulin resistance due to a weakening of signaling pathways.

Gut Microbiome, Obesity, and Insulin Resistance

Inflammation, which occurs with obesity, decreases insulin sensitivity. This causes a number of problems, and can lead to chronic complications because the body is not equipped to produce healthy, protective inflammation when invaded by antigens (Lee et al., 2019).

Weight loss can help significantly decrease cytokine buildup in the gut, which will help decrease inflammation. When your body is able to properly manage inflammation, its ability to respond to insulin also improves, as these pathways are no longer being damaged by chronic inflammation (Shen at al., 2012).

Through changes in your diet, you will be able to not only lose weight, but also promote better gut health, which both work to improve your insulin sensitivity.

Microbiome and Overall Health

Your gut microbiome fills a number of roles when it comes to your health. Not only does it protect you from pathogens, but it also boosts your immune system, synthesizes amino acids and vitamins that you can only receive from bacteria, and breaks down dangerous food compounds.

As discussed earlier, your gut health influences your overall health. Because of this, maintaining a balanced gut microbiome is key to keeping your gut happy and healthy so that it can perform its many jobs and communicate with other bodily systems. Maintaining good gut health will help keep you healthy, both physically and mentally. It can also play a significant role in your diabetes management, as insulin sensitivity tends to improve when you have a healthy gut that is not impacted by inflammation.

Regulating your gut microbiota will also help keep you from becoming overweight, as nutrition plays a key role in keeping a healthy gut and a healthy weight. But it works the other way around as well; maintaining a healthy weight through diet and exercise will keep your gut microbiota in check. Once you are able to develop healthier lifestyle habits, including nutrition and physical activity, maintaining proper gut health will get easier, and then the more you are able to maintain proper gut health, the easier it will be to keep off excess weight (Bull & Plummer, 2014).

Bacterial Overgrowth and Its Many Complications

The Mayo Clinic (2022) gives a detailed account of SIBO. Small intestinal bacterial overgrowth, or SIBO, can cause gastrointestinal issues such as diarrhea, indigestion, abdominal pain, and bloating, which can become chronic and stand in the way of your happiness and overall well-being. When left untreated, it can also lead to more serious complications such as kidney stones, osteoporosis, an inability to absorb vitamins and nutrients from food, which will then lead to malnutrition and various deficiencies.

A SIBO diagnosis is achieved by process of elimination, which can sometimes make it difficult or a lengthier process to detect. If you have any of the following symptoms that do not go away on their own, it's important to talk to your doctor about the possibility of SIBO.

- diarrhea

- bloating

- abdominal pain

- constipation

- gas

- malnutrition

- unexplained weight loss

- discomfort after eating

- unexplained loss of appetite

- nausea

SIBO is brought on when the small intestine, which is not meant to hold very much bacteria, develops a buildup of bacteria, which then becomes a breeding ground for even more bacteria to grow and remain stagnant. Factors that may put you at an increased risk of developing SIBO include the following.

- previous gastric or abdominal surgery.

- diabetes

- diverticulosis (bulging pouches within the small intestine)

- previous radiation therapy in the abdominal area

- previous injury or current physical abnormality to the small intestine

- gastrointestinal fistula

- current or previous cancer within the gastrointestinal system

- Crohn's disease

Part 2:
Gut Health Protocol

Chapter 4:

Restoring Your Gut's Natural

Balance

We've gone over why it is so important to maintain good gut health, and the various issues that may arise following a gut imbalance. Now how exactly do we work to restore the underlying causes of a gut imbalance so that we can minimize unwanted symptoms?

First, you will want to see your doctor to discuss your specific situation and steps that you can take to combat your challenges. There is also a protocol called the four R's that can help you restore your gut health naturally. The four R's refer to (Zaremba, 2021):

1. Remove, which is the first step in this process, refers to the removal of anything that may be triggering your gastrointestinal issues. This includes any foods in your current diet that your system is sensitive to. For most people, this will include the basics: processed foods, refined carbs, sugars, additives, alcohol, unhealthy fats (saturated and trans fats), and more. But this also means identifying any kind of food that you have a sensitivity to. Common examples of these potential foods are gluten and dairy.

2. Replace, which is the next step in the process, refers to coming up with foods to stand in for those that you have eliminated from your diet in the first step. These replacement foods should be anti-inflammatory, nutritious, and healing to your digestion. In reality, this step should be done at about the same time as the first step because you will need to have a game plan

for the foods that you are going to eat instead of the foods that you are stepping away from. These foods can be lean protein, fiber, fruits and vegetables, omega-3 fatty acids (such as salmon), anti-inflammatory spices and herbs (such as rosemary, turmeric, and garlic), and extra-virgin olive oil (which can replace butter in your cooking, and which also contains anti-inflammatory properties as well as many other health benefits). You may also potentially want to take dietary supplements such as digestive enzymes or bile acid supplements—your doctor can help you come up with a plan for which supplements will benefit you.

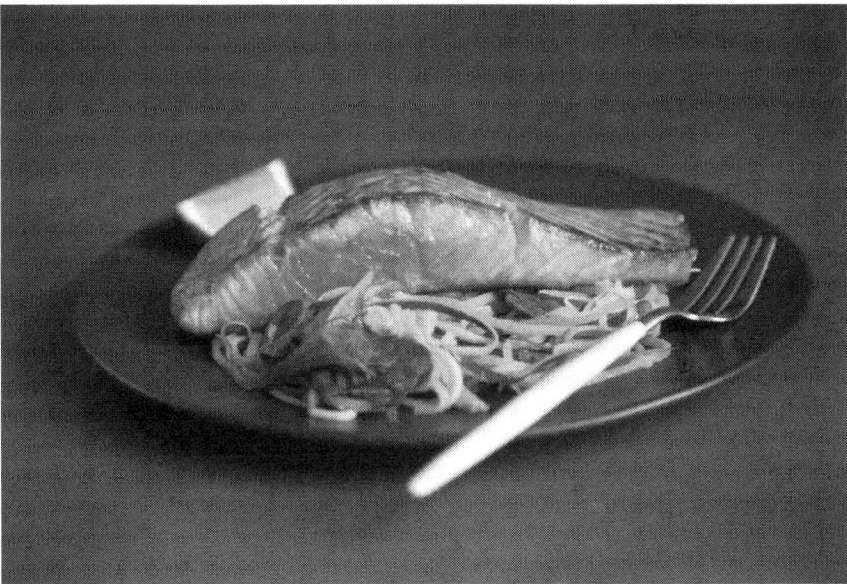

3. Re-inoculate, which is the third step in the process, refers to the reinforcement of the gut's microbiota. Here you will solidify your gut's balance by adding in probiotics to encourage the growth of healthy bacteria. There are many probiotic supplements that you can take, as well as probiotics that are naturally occurring in fermented foods.

4. Repair, which is the last step in the process, refers to the healing of the gut's wall. During this step, your diet will play a huge role in your gut's ability to rebuild the mucous membrane that protects your gut wall. Some foods and supplements that encourage gut wall regrowth include aloe vera, omega-3 fatty acids, vitamin D, zinc, and polyphenols.

The four R's are a great protocol to follow because they will help with a wide variety of underlying issues that may be causing your gut imbalance. Practicing the four R's will help alleviate your gastrointestinal symptoms and can make a huge difference in your health, happiness, and life!

Signs of Poor Gut Health

Poor gut health means that the bad bacteria has taken control over the good bacteria in your gut. A number of problems can arise from this. Here are some potential signs that you may have a gut imbalance (Nunez, 2022):

- trouble sleeping

- sugar cravings

- chronic fatigue

- unintentional weight fluctuations

- changes in mood, including irritability, depression, and anxiety

- autoimmune issues (i.e., thyroid problems, type 1 diabetes, arthritis)

- digestive problems (i.e., bloating, heartburn, ibs, diarrhea, constipation, irregular bowel movements)

- allergies

- skin issues (such as rashes, acne, or dandruff)

- headaches

- unexplained bad breath

- new food sensitivities

- inability to concentrate

An unhealthy diet is among the number one causes of gut problems. With an unhealthy diet that includes processed foods, additives, sugar, and unhealthy fats, unhealthy bacteria will thrive. On the other hand, with a healthy diet that is rich in fiber, plant foods, and other nutrients, the good bacteria in your gut will grow and thrive.

However, your diet is not the only potential contributing factor. Other factors that are beneficial to recognize include taking certain medications (like frequent use of antibiotics), chronic stress, unhealthy sleep habits, alcohol consumption, consuming foods that you have sensitivities to, and traveling.

Eating to Feed Those Microbiomes

It's important to identify the foods that are currently in your diet and working against your gut health, as well as the foods that you can replace them with so that you feed the good bacteria in your gut.

The microbiome diet is a new diet that is geared at achieving exactly this. Petre (2019) gives a detailed description of this diet. It can also help boost your metabolism, help with weight loss, and help get rid of sugar cravings.

The first step of the diet is to go through the four R's, which we discussed previously.

The second step of the diet is geared at giving your metabolism a boost through the food that you consume. This phase should last 28 days. After these 28 days, your gut health should be largely restored, which should give you some more flexibility with what you can eat while still maintaining good gut health. You will want to eat the new foods you have become familiar with that encourage gut health. Try to avoid any of the foods that you have identified as fuel for the bad bacteria in your gut about 90% of the time you eat. In doing so, you will be able to eat "cheat foods" in up to four meals per week. Don't go crazy with this though! Remember to eat these foods in moderation when you do have them. You should also be adding foods like dairy, legumes, eggs, and whole grains, back into your diet if you had previously removed them to identify any sensitivities.

The last phase of this diet is meant to be maintained long-term. Because sticking to intense diets is almost never something that is maintainable for most people, this diet proposes that after your 28 days in phase two, you can comply with the diet you have tailored for your gut health 70% of the time. This gives you the freedom to eat foods that you want but that may not necessarily fall into the good gut health category 30% of the time (or roughly one meal a day). However, with this 30% leeway, you should still practice eating in moderation and stay away from processed foods and foods with added sugars as much as you can manage. Hopefully, with the introduction of new foods, you will have fewer sugar cravings and find healthier foods that you are able to enjoy equally. And because you are eating less sugar overall, when you do allow yourself an occasional treat, you will likely not even want foods with as highly concentrated sugar levels as you had previously needed to feed your sugar cravings.

Foods that fuel your good gut bacteria are typically foods that contain rich nutrients and fiber. It is also recommended that you increase the variety of fruits and vegetables you consume so that you get a wider array of nutrients and vitamins. An easy and unexpected way to achieve this is by using more herbs and spices in your cooking. You can also start using different types of leafy greens in salads, as opposed to just one kind of lettuce every time you make a salad. Eating a variety of whole grains, nuts, legumes, and beans is also recommended so as to get a wider range of nutrients and health benefits. Doing this has the added benefit of making your meals even more tasty and interesting!

A general rule to follow is to add more (both quantity and variety) spices, herbs, fruits, vegetables, nuts, whole grains, beans, legumes, and fermented foods into your diet. Once you get comfortable experimenting with new foods, try setting a goal to eat 30 different plant foods per week (O'Connor, 2022). You can start by keeping a food journal to track what kinds and how many plant foods you are already eating. While 30 different plant foods may seem like a lot, you may be already closer to this number than you think! Writing out the plant foods that you are eating can help encourage you to stay on track. Also, remember that plant foods aren't just fruits and vegetables. This category also includes herbs, spices, and nuts—anything that comes from plants!

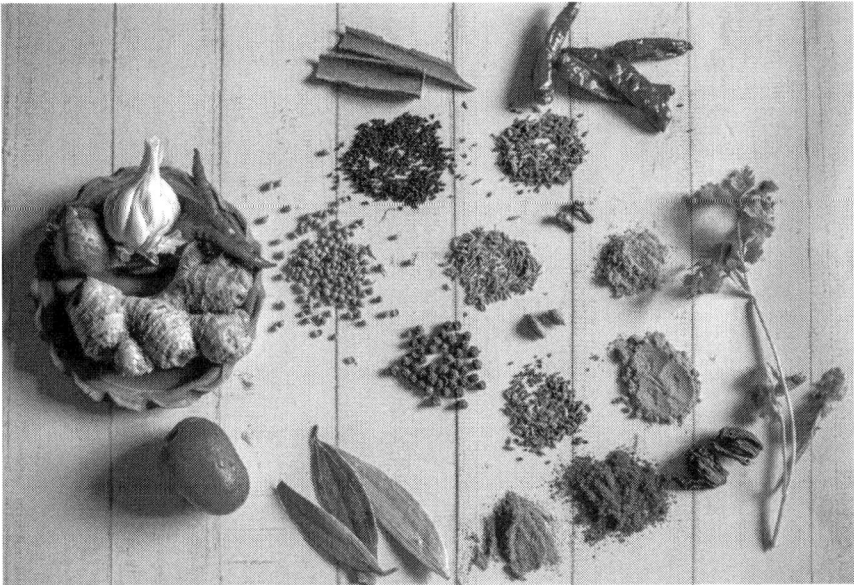

How to Maintain the Microbiome

Once you've achieved your ideal gut microbiota, maintaining it is up to you. Eating healthy foods while staying away from your old unhealthy eating habits is key for maintaining good gut health, but there are other steps you can take to make sure your gut stays happy.

Eating a plant-based diet is helpful for a lot of people. With a plant-based diet, you are consuming mainly foods that come from plants. This will ensure that you receive lots of fiber, and when the fiber passes through your digestive system, the good bacteria in your gut "break down the plant polysaccharides through fermentation into short-chain fatty acids, the largest amount as butyrate," which is what the cells in your colon ideally want to use for energy (Bachus, 2018, para. 1). This process promotes gut health and will also help prevent colon cancer.

Eating different fermented foods once daily will help maintain the good bacteria in your gut, as they add more good bacteria. This way, you are helping to ensure that the good bacteria in your gut will never become overrun by the bad bacteria. Try setting a goal to consume one to two servings per day of fermented food. Remember, the more variety of fermented foods you can bring into your diet, the better, as different foods will bring along different health benefits and nutrients.

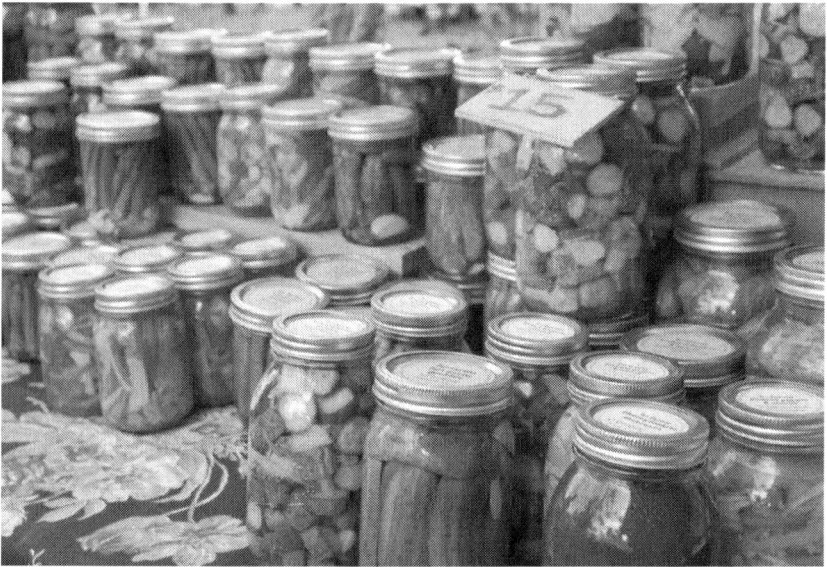

Incorporating polyphenols in your diet is also a great way to combat inflammation while encouraging the growth of good bacteria and preventing the growth of harmful bacteria. Polyphenols can be found in foods such as blueberries, cherries, green tea, pomegranates, and dark chocolate (just don't overdo it on the dark chocolate) (Bachus, 2018).

Dark chocolate, however, is actually a great substitute for a sweeter treat that you may have more regularly indulged in before changing your eating habits. As discussed before, it's not about pledging to never have anything sweet ever again—this is both unrealistic and not exactly necessary. Rather, you should limit the sugars that you consume and also cut back on added sugars that are highly concentrated in unhealthy and over-processed foods. The more you are able to do this, the less you will want those ultra-sugary foods to begin with. Some foods that you can have as a sweet treat and that provide benefits for your gut include dark chocolate, fruits, sweet potatoes, honey, and coconut flour.

Don't overdo it on antibiotics. While antibiotics are sometimes needed to help fight off sickness, you should only take them when absolutely needed. This is because, while they are used to fight off bad bacteria that make you sick, they also kill helpful bacteria. When you do have to take an antibiotic, talk to your doctor about taking a supplement such as Saccharomyces boulardii, which can help restore the good bacteria in your gut even when antibiotics are present. Another tactic is doubling down on your probiotic and prebiotic intake following antibiotic use (Bachus, 2018).

Cut out red meat. So many meat farms raise their animals with antibiotics, which stay in your food and get into your own system upon consumption. By cutting back on (or cutting out) red meat, you reduce the amount of antibiotics that can easily find their way into your system and kill off the good bacteria in your gut. Also, by taking on a plant-based diet, you are likely to consume more fiber, which helps the good bacteria in your gut flourish (Canadian Digestive Health Foundation, 2022).

Maintain a sleep schedule. When you sleep at irregular times or wake up throughout the night without allowing your body to go through a complete sleep cycle, the microbiota in your gut become disrupted as well. When this happens, you are at greater risk for developing issues like inflammation (Canadian Digestive Health Foundation, 2022).

Exercise and maintain a physically active lifestyle. Exercise helps maintain good gut health. This can be as simple as taking a half-hour walk. Increasing activity in your daily life can make all the difference to your gut microbiota (Canadian Digestive Health Foundation, 2022).

Natural Ways to Improve Gut Health

There are so many ways that you can take charge of your gut health. Here are some steps to naturally improve your gut health (Leonard, 2019):

- Increase your probiotic and fermented foods intake.

  - Consuming more probiotics will help boost your gut's good bacteria. You can take a probiotic supplement, or you can also eat more fermented foods, which are natural probiotics. If taking a probiotic supplement (just as with any supplement), make sure you consult with your doctor first.

- Increase your prebiotic fiber intake.

  - Prebiotic fiber is like fuel for the probiotics in your system. Consuming prebiotics will help encourage the growth of healthy bacteria in your gut.

- Consume less sugar and sweeteners.

- Reduce stress.

- Limit antibiotic use.

- Exercise.

- Improve your sleep quality.

- Quit smoking.

- Eat more plant-based foods.

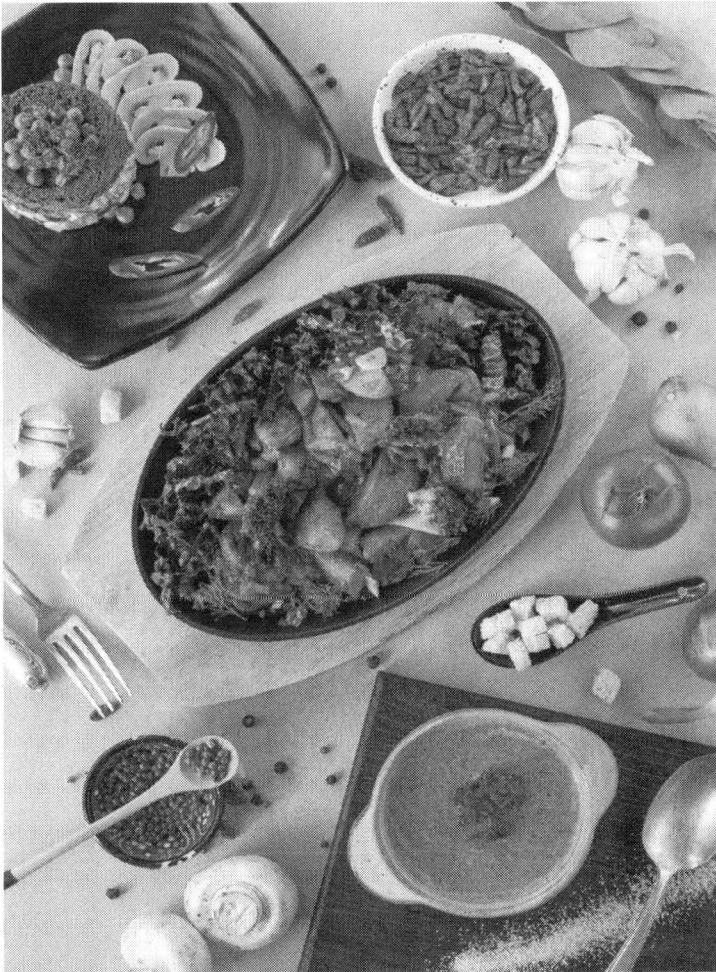

- Adopt a vegetarian diet.

- Keep variety in your diet.

- Drink water throughout the day.

- Increase your polyphenol intake.

The Influence of Probiotics on Gut Microbiota

Probiotics help balance your gut microbiome, which in turn provides you with many different health benefits, including better protection against pathogens through a strengthened immune system and gut wall. The immune system and gut microbiota are strongly linked, and when we increase our probiotic intake, we are taking steps to ensure that our gut microbiota is properly balanced. With this balance comes increased immunity. The relationship between intestinal flora, immunity, and probiotics is important to our overall health and well-being (Wang et al., 2021).

Chapter 5:

The Holistic Nutrition Solution

Holistic healing often begins the best in the gut. Naturopathic medicine works quite effectively when applied to gut health, as your gut health is largely influenced by the types of food you eat and other natural factors. Specific issues that are managed quite successfully through naturopathic medicine include ulcerative colitis, Crohn's disease, IBS, food intolerances, liver disease, diverticulosis/diverticulitis, gallbladder dysfunction, GERD and gastritis, peptic ulcer disease, and small intestine bacterial overgrowth (SIBO). If you have any of these conditions, naturopathic medicine may be a great option for you to begin to implement in your day-to-day life (Richmond Natural Medicine, n.d.).

What exactly is naturopathic medicine? It follows the Hippocratic philosophy that "all disease begins in the gut." Even if you do not have one of the conditions mentioned above, naturopathic medicine can help almost everyone, as it is a holistic practice that can bring about positive change in a wide range of areas. Because the gut is so intricately linked to many other areas concerning both physical and mental health, often when people use naturopathic medicine to aid their gut health, they see improvement in a variety of other areas of their overall health.

When the body is taken care of, it has a natural ability to heal. Most frequently, there are a number of issues at hand because the body is so interconnected. Because of this, it is common to approach naturopathic healing with a layered approach, as opposed to simply implementing one change. A layered approach leads to longer-lasting results, as all areas of concern will be addressed rather than just one. Addressing only one issue would leave you needing to address lingering problems.

Since no two people will ever have the exact same thing going on in their bodies, it is beneficial to take on the mindset that you need to work out what's specifically going on in your body and what your body needs to heal. It is essential during this time to remember to be patient with yourself. This will take some time to figure out. For instance, if you are dealing with food sensitivity, you will need to try cutting out certain types of food from your diet one by one before being able to identify your sensitivity. Because of this, an approach that works for one person may not work for the next, and this is perfectly normal.

Does the SIBO Diet Work?

SIBO is a common condition for people with an unhealthy gut, as it is characterized by an overgrowth of bad bacteria in the small intestine. The SIBO diet is geared at tackling this issue naturally, and it is often highly effective. Because of this, it can offer a good alternative to antibiotics. However, you will want to speak to your doctor about this plan of action to see if it is a good option for your specific situation as opposed to antibiotics (Ruscio, 2022).

The SIBO diet is typically quite effective, both when used alone or in addition to another form of treatment under doctor supervision.

When starting out on the diet, you will want to keep it simple. Keeping your meals on the simpler side will help you figure out what works and what doesn't in your diet. You will also want to repeat meals as necessary in the beginning. Once you get a better feel for which types of food agree with you and which don't, you can start to branch out and add a wider variety of foods to your diet.

Be prepared for changes to happen. You may experience psychological changes such as mood shifts. When your gut is inflamed, it is common for this inflammation to travel to the brain, and when this happens, changes in your neurotransmitters are likely. It is best to keep this in the back of your mind so that if you experience mood changes, it does not come as a surprise, and you will be better prepared to manage symptoms.

Whichever variation of the diet you are following, be sure to really stick to it. This will make it the most effective for you so that you will be able to more quickly see results.

If the diet does not seem to be working for you after a few weeks, you may want to consider trying a new approach.

When you start introducing new foods into your diet, make sure to do so slowly. Adding in one type of new food at a time is the best way to recognize any potential changes in your body that this type of food causes. Make sure to really pay close attention to how your body changes (or does not change) with the introduction of one specific food at a time, for two days following the introduction. If you do not notice any changes in your body after these two days, you can introduce another new type of food into your diet a few days after this.

If you follow these strategies as part of your diet management, the SIBO diet is likely to provide you with positive and informative results. Now let's get into the different subcategories of the SIBO diet.

The Different Types of SIBO Diet

There are a number of variations on the SIBO diet depending on your specific needs. However, all of the variations have an element that focuses on reducing carbohydrate intake so as to reduce the fuel for bacteria to continue to grow. Let's take a look at the different variations of the SIBO diet.

Low-FODMAP Diet

Tchiki Davis (n.d.) provides a detailed explanation of the low-FODMAP diet. This diet significantly reduces the carbohydrates that feed bacteria. Specifically, it eliminates fermentable oligosaccharides, disaccharides, monosaccharides, and polyols (FODMAPs)—five different categories of naturally occurring sugars—from your diet. The aim here is to reduce SIBO and IBS symptoms (i.e., bloating, diarrhea, gas, pain in the gut area, and constipation) by taking out these types of foods from your diet. Some examples of foods that are high in FODMAP content are

- dairy

- dried fruit

- sweeteners

- cauliflower, cabbage, and broccoli

- prebiotic fiber

- beans and lentils

- wheat

These types of foods are not easily digested in the beginning area of the small intestine. Because of this, they can travel through the rest of the small intestine without breaking down. When this happens, the food pieces also draw water along with them, which can cause cramping and bloating. Once they reach the large intestine, they feed the bacteria here. This feeding process tends to produce a lot of gas, which can be uncomfortable. Other symptoms of sensitivity to FODMAP foods include constipation, diarrhea, fatigue, and mood changes. Switching to a low-FODMAP diet can help tremendously with alleviating these symptoms.

When starting the low-FODMAP diet, you will want to eliminate foods that are high in FODMAP content. Then, you will want to reintroduce these foods slowly and one at a time (by sugar category). By the end of this process, you will be able to identify which of these foods were causing your unwanted symptoms. In the long term, you can avoid only the foods that you found to be problematic for your body, while keeping the other FODMAP foods that your body did not have issues with.

SCD Diet

For people who need a bit more than the low-FODMAP diet, the specific carbohydrate diet (SCD) is a more aggressive approach to the carb-restrictive diet. With this diet, you will be removing all grains and complex carbohydrates in order to help reduce your unwanted gastrointestinal symptoms. This diet is recommended for those who saw some improvement with the low-FODMAP diet, but who still need to reduce their symptoms further (Ruscio, 2020).

On this diet, you will get rid of sugars, grains, and starchy vegetables. However, you may still eat simple sugars and fruits and vegetables with simple sugars. This diet is also highly effective for people with celiac disease and people with inflammatory bowel diseases like Crohn's.

Cedars Sinai Diet

This diet is used to limit the growth of bacteria through the use of limiting fermentable foods. On this diet, you will eliminate snacking in order to give 4-5 hours of non-eating space between meals. The following are other actions required by the diet:

- Cut out sugar additives, including sugar-free sweeteners.

- Drink at least eight cups of water per day.

- Limit beans, peas, soy, yogurt, lentils, and other high-residue foods.

- Limit leafy greens, cauliflower, broccoli, cabbage, and brussels sprouts.

- Consume cooked vegetables daily (cooked vegetables are easier to digest than raw), avoiding vegetables from the bullet above.

- Consume protein from fish, poultry, and eggs.

- Consume ½-1 cup of carbs per meal. In this case, you will want to choose foods like white pasta, white rice, and white bread over their whole-grain alternatives.

- Only eat whole fruits, and limit consumption to two servings per day. Avoid bananas, pears, and apples.

- Cut out dairy and soy. You can opt instead for options like unsweetened coconut or rice milk.

- Try to avoid coffee, tea, or any other caffeinated beverages as much as possible. If you do need caffeine, choose tea, and only drink it in moderation.

- Maintain moderate physical activity and consume the amount of calories best suited to your needs (you should discuss this with your doctor to find out how many calories you should be aiming for per day.)

Elemental Diet

This diet is an option for people whose bodies do not respond to changes in their diet. The elemental diet is meant to be used in the short term, either just before starting a diet to tackle SIBO symptoms or on its own for two to three weeks. It can, however, be utilized in the long term as well. When implementing this diet for a longer period of time, it is recommended that you only use it to replace one meal per day (Davis, n.d.).

This diet replaces your regular meals with a complete nutrition liquid replacement. In doing this, you are eliminating any potential fuel for existing harmful bacteria in your gut. You are also allowing your digestive system time to relax from potentially strenuous digestive processes that may be causing inflammation and other issues.

Paleo Diet

The idea behind this diet is to only eat foods that were available to early humans (during the Paleolithic Era). This includes vegetables, fruits, lean meats, seafood, seeds, nuts, and eggs. Dairy products, grains, and legumes are not included in this diet, as humans during this time did not yet have access to these types of foods (Mayo Clinic Staff, 2020).

This diet is commonly used to lose weight or maintain a healthy weight, improve blood pressure and cholesterol, reduce triglycerides, and reduce risks such as cardiovascular disease. It helps with these target areas by also cutting out added salt, added sugars, starchy vegetables such as white potatoes or corn, and processed foods.

Biphasic Diet

This diet draws from elements of the low-FODMAP diet and the SCD. Its aim is to have a bit more structure than the other two diets, while still tackling the same objectives. The diet is broken up into two phases in order to limit any potential side effects, including fungal and bacterial die-off. However, it aims to manage bacterial growth in the small intestine at the same time (Essential Stacks, 2022).

During phase one, referred to as the reduce and repair phase (four to six weeks), foods are put in one of three categories—"restricted diet," "semi-restricted," or "avoid." When starting, you will want to only use foods from the restricted diet category. Depending on your improvement, people may begin adding in foods from the semi-restricted category as early as the first week.

During phase two, referred to as the remove and restore phase (four to six weeks), foods are put into one of two categories—"phase two diet," or "avoid." All of the foods that you could eat during phase one are also allowed during this phase. In addition, you may also begin to add in other foods like potatoes.

Low Histamine Diet

Osborn (2020) details the low histamine diet and its uses. Histamines are a type of chemical that our bodies naturally produce; however, histamines are also in certain foods, which some people have negative reactions to, including gastrointestinal issues. A low histamine diet is a type of elimination diet that usually lasts about four weeks. The goal is that after these four weeks, you should be able to recognize which foods trigger a histamine-intolerant reaction in your body. Then, you can avoid these foods moving forward.

Foods that can be part of the elimination process include the following

- cured meats

- alcohol

- eggplant

- tomatoes

- spinach

- canned, salted, or frozen fish

- vinegar

- fermented foods

GAPS Diet

This diet is designed for people whose gut health has been more seriously damaged. In this case, a SIBO diet (such as the low-FODMAP diet) is used in combination with this diet—either simultaneously or before starting the GAPS diet so that your SIBO is cleared away first. The GAPS diet is designed to treat gastrointestinal conditions like SIBO and IBS, and also neurological conditions such as depression, anxiety, and ADHD.

On the GAPS diet, you will go through six phases that will help rebuild your gut wall and overall gut health. During each phase, you will add in more foods to your diet. This diet is recommended only for those with more serious and multi-layered gut issues. It is also recommended that you consult your doctor before going on this diet, and especially important that you work with a doctor or nutritionist if you are using the GAPS diet while you still have SIBO symptoms.

Acceptable Foods in a Low FODMAP Diet

Here are some commonly-enjoyed foods (by category) that adhere to the low-FODMAP diet (IBS Diets, 2022).

Vegetables

- alfalfa

- broccoli

- carrots

- bok choy

- bean sprouts

- green beans

- cucumber

- bell peppers

- tomato

- lettuce

- broccolini

- cabbage

- chives

- collard greens
- eggplant
- ginger
- kale
- potatoes
- zucchini
- ginger
- turnips
- parsnips
- tomato
- pumpkin
- spaghetti squash

Fruit

- grapes
- banana
- blueberries
- oranges
- cantaloupe
- honeydew
- grapefruit
- lemon

- lime
- papaya
- kiwi
- strawberries
- sranberries
- raspberries
- coconut
- guava
- pineapple
- passion fruit

Meat and meat substitutes (make sure that everything is fresh and without additives)

- chicken
- tuna
- cod
- salmon
- trout
- haddock
- crab
- shrimp
- oysters
- lobster

- mussels
- eggs
- turkey
- beef
- pork
- quorn meat substitute
- lamb
- chorizo
- tempeh
- tofu

Dairy and dairy substitutes

- brie
- cheddar
- feta
- camembert
- almond milk
- oat milk
- coconut milk
- swiss
- mozzarella
- parmesan

- goat cheese
- Monterey jack cheese

Grains and nuts

- oats
- quinoa
- corn flour
- potato flour
- polenta
- rice cakes
- rice crackers
- tortilla chips
- gluten-free products
- rice
- corn tortillas
- buckwheat
- bulgur
- corn bread
- almonds
- brazil nuts
- chestnuts
- Hazelnuts

- macadamia nuts
- peanuts
- pine nuts
- walnuts
- pumpkin seeds

Herbs, spices, and oils

- basil
- sage
- coriander
- cilantro
- bay leaves
- mint
- oregano
- parsley
- thyme
- tarragon
- rosemary
- curry leaves
- lemongrass
- black pepper
- cardamon

- all spice
- cumin
- curry powder
- fennel seeds
- nutmeg
- paprika
- saffron
- turmeric
- cinnamon
- chipotle chili powder
- cloves
- mustard seeds
- star anise
- avocado oil
- coconut oil
- olive oil
- sesame oil
- sunflower oil
- peanut oil
- canola oil
- vegetable oil

Benefits of the SIBO Diet

The SIBO diet has the potential to bring tremendous relief to your gastrointestinal system. It can not only help strengthen your gut microbiota and gut wall, but it can also help relieve unwanted symptoms of SIBO that get in the way of your daily life and happiness, such as painful bloating, gas, constipation, and diarrhea.

Additionally, you will gain the knowledge of what kinds of foods your body responds to well versus what it cannot tolerate. Moving forward, you will be able to tailor your diet to fit these needs while still maintaining a variety of foods in your diet that provide you with a variety of nutrients. In fact, the SIBO diet—though limiting at first—can actually help bring more nutrients into your diet because it encourages a wider variety of the types of food that your body can tolerate. Lots of people have nutritional deficiencies without even realizing it; this is because many people tend to eat the same foods without branching out and bringing in a wider variety of foods into their diet. In this way, the SIBO diet can address any potential nutrient deficiencies that you may have previously had.

How It Helps With the Management of IBS

Following the SIBO diet, your gut will have a more balanced bacterial life because the diet will get rid of an overgrowth of bacteria in your gut that has been contributing to your gastrointestinal symptoms. It will also help prevent the existing bacteria in your gut from multiplying further. You will also experience less inflammation, which is a cause of many unwanted and painful gastrointestinal symptoms, including IBS.

Dos and Don'ts of an IBS Diet

Do

- Eat smaller meals more frequently.

- Slow down the pace of your eating.

- Avoid foods that are tough to digest or overstimulating (large meals, high-fat content).

- Eat breakfast.

- Keep a food journal and try eliminating foods that you notice have a pattern of upsetting your gut.

- Eliminate foods one-at-a-time to best identify how these foods affect your body.

- Consume soluble fiber such as

    - root vegetables

    - oatmeal

    - most fruits

Don't

- Consume caffeine

- Consume insoluble fiber such as

    - whole grains

    - eggplant

    - corn

    - green beans

    - leafy greens

    - broccoli

    - strawberries

    - blueberries

- raisins

- pineapple

- raspberries

- kiwi

- Consume dairy

- Consume fried foods

- Consume added sugars or sweeteners, including sugar-free sweeteners

Should You Consider Probiotics?

Consuming both probiotics and prebiotics will help maintain good gut health. Prebiotics are actually the good bacteria's ideal source for energy—the indigestible fibers that they receive from plant-derived foods. Probiotics will help spread good bacteria to your digestive tract. However, if you have SIBO or similar problems, you will want to talk to your doctor before taking probiotics. This way, your doctor can work with you to come up with a plan that best suits you. You and your doctor may want to address the issue of bad bacteria buildup—potentially through antibiotics, for example—before working to build your good bacteria.

Chapter 6:

Combating Inflammation and

Insulin Resistance

When we hear about inflammation, it is usually used to describe harmful and even painful symptoms. However, there are two types of inflammation: the good and the bad. Good inflammation—also called acute inflammation—actually helps keep us healthy! It is triggered by our immune system and works to defend the body from things like pathogens, toxins, and physical sharp objects. When these types of harmful foreign bodies invade our bodies, acute inflammation helps restore the affected body part.

When your immune system senses a harmful foreign substance in your body, it activates acute inflammation. During this process, white blood cells travel to the affected area and cytokines (a type of compound substance) are released in the area. The white blood cells and cytokines work together to attack the invading antigen. When the foreign substance is a physical puncture causing an injury, the cytokines and white blood cells help stop further damage to the surrounding tissue and help clot the blood around the area to prevent further bleeding. When the damage is at a controlled level, white blood cells will work to repair the damage and start to push out any lingering debris. This results in symptoms that may include redness, pain, pus, fever, and swelling, or inflammation. Since this type of inflammation is acute, these symptoms both come and go relatively quickly (Rocky Mountain Analytical, n.d.).

The benefit lies in the body's ability to quickly attack the antigen. The key here is that once the antigen is defeated, the inflammation goes away—hence, the acute aspect. The quick nature of the acute inflammation process allows the body's immune system sufficient downtime. This allows the body's immune response the ability to come back in full swing the next time it is needed.

When acute inflammation occurs, other cells that are not involved but that happen to be near the affected area will be damaged by the attacking white blood cells and cytokines. This is a normal part of the process—collateral damage if you will. When this happens, the effects are quite minor and the body is not impacted in any significant manner. However, the more inflammation, the more collateral damage to your healthy cells. This is part of the reason why chronic inflammation is so damaging to the body.

That brings us to bad inflammation—chronic inflammation. This is when the inflammation process does not resolve itself in a timely manner. Instead, it lingers because either the issue at hand is not being quickly resolved or because the body is unnecessarily triggering the inflammatory response, which can be due to a number of different factors.

With chronic inflammation, the immune system does not get its downtime to rest, and because of this, it is not always able to attack invading antigens at its full capacity. When this happens, our whole body suffers. We may not realize it, but we are exposed to antigens every day, all the time. Antigens range from small cuts or scrapes to germs that cause the common cold.

Chronic inflammation throws our whole immune system off balance. Once this is the case, the body may react by triggering inflammation that does not align with the problem at hand. You may get inflammation that is triggered by what seems to be the smallest things. This is because your immune system is misreading the threat level. Things like low-level toxins that may be present in food and water, not getting enough sleep, stress, inflammatory foods, and physical inactivity can all suddenly become huge triggers for inflammation.

What's more is that since the immune system is so closely linked to other bodily systems, such as the endocrine and nervous systems, when you have chronic inflammation, these other systems can start to become dysregulated as well. The further dysregulated various other connected systems get, the harder it becomes to get everything back on track, as the issue has, at this point, become quite multi-faceted. This can also trigger certain genes that you are predisposed to, such as autoimmune conditions like type 1 diabetes.

Sugar and Starch: Their Link to Inflammation

As we discussed earlier, inflammation is not necessarily a bad thing. It is naturally-occurring, and can actually help the body if the immune system is able to maintain its proper function. Certain foods may trigger some inflammation in the body as well. This is normal and does not mean that anything is wrong with your body or that these foods necessarily need to be completely cut out of your diet. However, eating such foods in excess may cause prolonged inflammation, which can lead to chronic inflammation—and that is something we don't want.

Sugar is a food that causes inflammation, so when eaten in excessive amounts or when eaten frequently, chronic inflammation in the body may occur. Particularly for those who do not know about inflammatory foods, consuming excessive sugar can be dangerous because they may also be eating sugar in combination with other inflammatory foods. A diet that causes chronic inflammation can lead to more serious health issues, including cancer, heart disease, allergies, and diabetes.

Sugar, inflammation, and diabetes are all interlinked. Sugar can lead to inflammation, which can lead to insulin resistance, which can bring on type 1 diabetes. Sugar can also lead to obesity, which can lead to type 2 diabetes.

Refined starches, such as white bread, white flour, white pasta, white rice, sodas, cereals, and pastries, are similarly associated with inflammation. In fact, they have very similar effects on the body as added sugars. These kinds of starches spike blood sugar levels, bring about weight gain, and make the body more resistant to insulin as well.

Sugar and starch lead to chronic inflammation in a number of ways. To start, they make your body produce an excessive amount of advanced glycation end products (AGEs), which are compounds made when fat, sugar, and protein enter the bloodstream. When you have too many of these compounds in your bloodstream, you get inflammation.

Sugar and starch also destroy your gut wall. When this happens, toxins can easily go straight through the gut wall and into your bloodstream, which can also cause inflammation.

These foods also contain LDL cholesterol, which is linked to C-reactive protein. With an excess amount of LDL cholesterol and C-reactive protein, you get inflammation.

As mentioned previously, these foods are also linked to weight gain. When you have an unhealthy amount of body fat, you may experience insulin resistance and inflammation.

Strategies to Put an End to Your Sugar Addiction

Overcoming a sugar addiction can seem like an overwhelming challenge when you first look at it. However, the best way to start is by breaking it down. You don't have to do a total 360 overnight. Here are some steps that you can take to make this challenge more manageable.

For starters, eat regular meals. Don't try to skip meals to compensate for all the sugar you've been consuming. Also remember not to skip breakfast! Many people feel rushed in the mornings and end up disregarding this extremely important meal. If this situation rings true to you, try to stock your fridge with quick and easy breakfast foods, or prepare your breakfast ahead of time. It is always a great move to have some protein in your breakfast, as this will help you feel fuller for longer. Stay away from the many sugar-packed and highly-processed breakfast foods that you'll see in the grocery store.

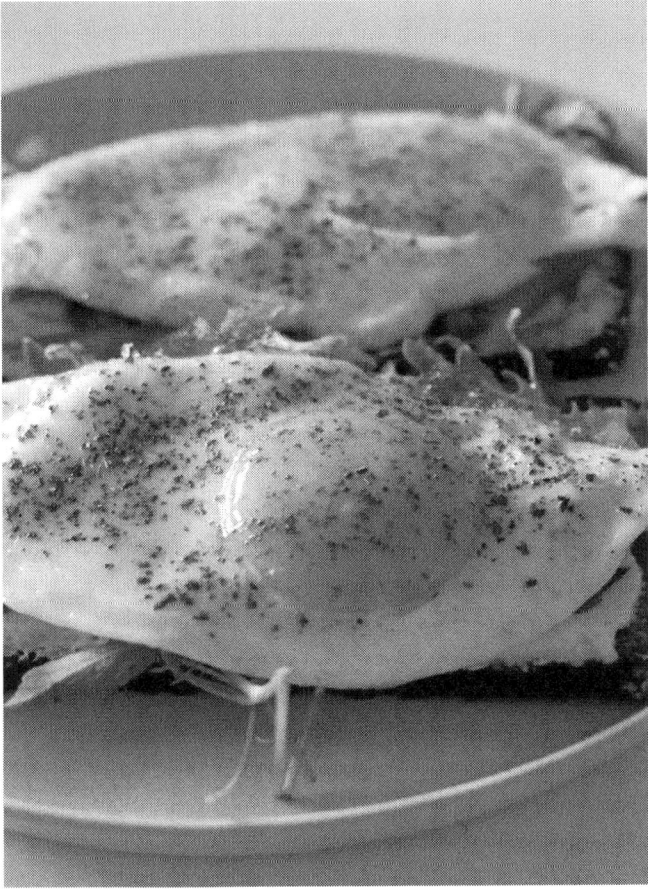

When you are full, you are less likely to crave sugar. On the other hand, when you do not eat regularly and are often hungry, this means that your blood sugar levels are dropping, and as a result your body will crave sugar. When you do experience this, it is helpful to remember that, although you may feel like your body is craving sugar, there are much better ways to go about bringing your blood sugar back up to a healthy level. Eating a non-sugary meal or snack will help you manage your blood sugar and will also allow you to remain clear-headed, as opposed to feeling weakened by your sugar cravings.

When you go for a meal or a snack, try to choose whole foods. The more naturally-occurring the food, the less processed it is, and the less processed it is, the less additives it will contain, including added sugars.

Also make sure that you are getting nutrients in every meal. Adding variety to your foods will help with this as well.

Making sure you stay hydrated throughout the day will also help curb your sugar cravings. Keeping a reusable water bottle on hand will help remind you to drink water, as well as remind you to choose water instead of purchasing a sugary drink, such as soda or juice. Unfortunately, sometimes our brains unintentionally trick us into thinking we are hungry when what we actually are is thirsty. Sipping on water throughout the day will help prevent this from happening in the first place, but if it does happen, you can drink some water to see if you are actually just thirsty.

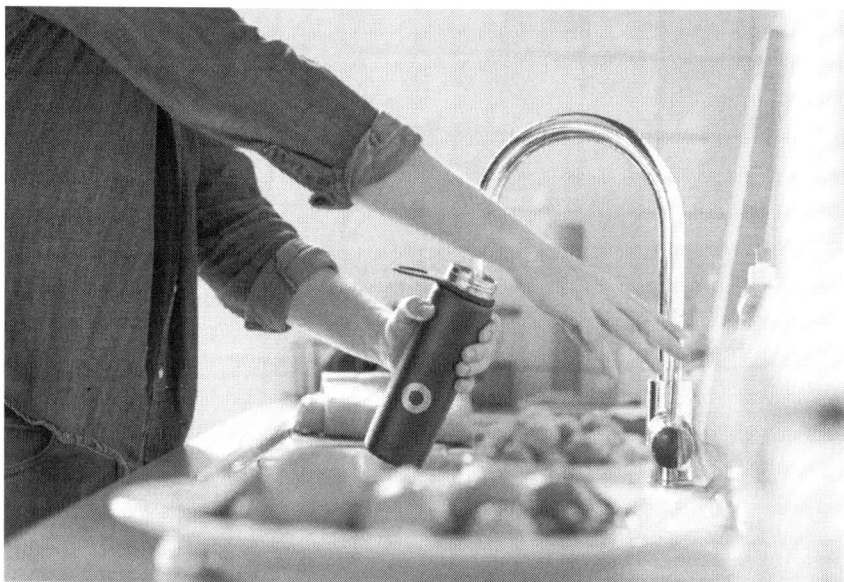

It can also be helpful to think of your new diet not as limiting certain foods but as adding other types of foods. This reframing allows you to think in the positive, rather than the negative, which will help keep you motivated and get you excited about your new diet. Additionally, thinking about and also experiencing how much better you feel when you eat foods that nourish you rather than harm you is a great way to frame your diet in a positive light.

Finally, be kind to yourself. Vowing never to eat sugar again is unrealistic and will only lead to disappointment when you do inevitably have a sweet treat. It is much more effective to practice moderation. Allow yourself to indulge in sugary snacks for special occasions, and when you do so, practice moderation with the quantity of your servings. It can also help to choose the sugary foods that you do want to indulge in from time to time while identifying those that you can get rid of. Think about all the foods that you would not consider to be "sweets," but that are actually extremely sugary. For instance, ketchup tends to have extremely high sugar content, but you likely aren't even aware of the amount of sugar you are consuming when you do eat ketchup. This can be a non-"sweet" sugary food that you can give up more easily than, let's say, the occasional ice cream. When you do have a slip up, don't beat yourself up about it. Rather, move forward positively.

The Long-Term Complications of Inflammation

Systemic chronic inflammation (SCI) describes the "bad" kind of inflammation that lingers in the body in the long term. Contributing factors of SCI include lifestyle factors such as diet, sedentary lifestyle, and stress, as well as environmental factors such as air pollution. Recognizing these potential contributing factors is an important first step in changing the factors that you have control over. This is the best way to avoid long-term effects of SCI, including cancer, cardiovascular disease, diabetes, liver and kidney diseases, and other various neurodegenerative and autoimmune problems (El Camino Health, 2022).

SCI is a leading contributor in diseases worldwide. Actually, it is "recognized as the most significant cause of death in the world today, with more than 50% of all deaths being attributable to inflammation-related diseases" (Furman et al., 2019, para. 2). Even so, many people are not aware of how drastic inflammation can be when left untreated.

In addition to these more life-threatening risk factors of chronic inflammation, it can also play a significant role in your daily life. SCI makes the body go into what is referred to as "sickness behaviors," which is characterized by fatigue, depression, reduced libido, changes in sleep patterns, social withdrawal, insulin resistance, and heightened blood pressure. Your body goes into this mode in order to save energy, as inflammation uses significant energy, and chronic inflammation does not allow your body's immune system time to rejuvenate. Over long periods of time, all of these symptoms of SCI can not only take a toll on your overall health and well-being, but also significantly impact your quality of life.

The Link Between Insulin Resistance and Inflammation

Chronic inflammation can lead to increased insulin resistance. The collateral damage that your surrounding tissue and cells suffer from inflammation becomes significantly damaging to your body, as opposed to acute inflammation, where this collateral damage does not significantly impact your body. During SCI, your organs also suffer damage, which can lead to serious issues as well over time.

Even if you already have an existing health issue such as diabetes, the presence of SCI can drastically push the progression of the disease. Additionally, the presence of SCI weakens your immune system when it comes time to perform acute inflammation. Since the immune system is overworked, it cannot protect against antigens as well as it should. As a result, the body becomes more susceptible to infections and less responsive to vaccinations.

What is an Anti-Inflammatory Diet?

The good news is, you can drastically help regulate chronic inflammation through changes in your diet. An anti-inflammatory diet is largely plant-based, meaning that a majority of the foods you will eat come from plants. This includes vegetables, fruits, whole grains, spices, and herbs. The diet also encourages the consumption of lean proteins, omega-3 fatty acids, antioxidants, and healthy fats. By adding more (both in quantity and variety) of these types of food into your diet, you are encouraged to also limit or get rid of processed foods, sugars, alcohol, and red meat (Fletcher, 2022).

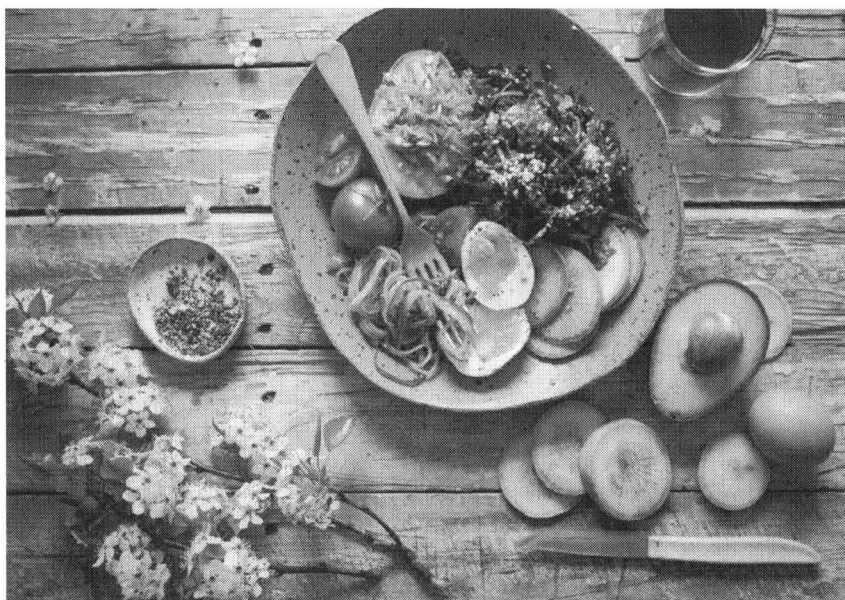

Those are the basic guidelines for an anti-inflammatory diet. However, many different diets adhere to these guidelines. Because of this, you have a variety of options when looking at specific diets to follow. You also do not necessarily have to follow one specific diet if you are able to follow these guidelines on your own.

As with any diet, you should consult your doctor before making significant changes to your diet so that you can work together to come up with a plan that best suits your needs and goals. Remember that everyone is different, and a diet that works great for one individual may not be as successful for another. Pay attention to your body, and if something isn't working, change it!

The Mediterranean diet and the DASH diet are two of the most widely-used and successful diets that fall into this category. Both of these diets are largely plant-based and have been proven to significantly reduce the effects of inflammation. They also have the added benefit of being easier to maintain in the long term. Rather than taking an aggressively limiting approach, these diets replace the unhealthy foods that you may currently be eating with healthier options. By focusing on what you can eat, rather than giving you unrealistically strict guidelines of foods you need to cut out of your diet for good, you are able to truly enjoy the new foods you are bringing into your diet. This way, you can focus on feeling holistically good, both physically and mentally, instead of constantly worrying about what you can and cannot eat.

The Mediterranean vs. the DASH Diet

These two diets actually have a lot of similarities, and they both adhere to an anti-inflammatory diet. Many people look at these two diets and struggle to choose one. However, you don't necessarily need to limit yourself to either one or the other. In fact, you can take key aspects from both diets and use them in your diet. It's all about figuring out what kind of dietary plan works best for you. These two diets are a great place to start, as they offer a wide variety of foods, unlike many fad diets that are extremely limiting and unsustainable in the long term.

The Mediterranean diet is based on different cultural diets around the Mediterranean. The diet developed around the '50s and '60s when researchers began looking into the relationship between cultural diets, longevity, and heart disease. During this time, researchers discovered that, on average, populations around the Mediterranean lived longer and had fewer instances of heart disease.

The Mediterranean diet consists mainly of plant-based foods that are naturally found in these regions, such as fruits, legumes, olives and olive oil, nuts, vegetables, and grains. Dairy, seafood, and poultry are also included in moderation. On this diet, you will eat foods that contain healthy fats, as healthy fats have health benefits such as reducing inflammation, cholesterol, and risks of heart disease and obesity.

Foods to eat liberally on the Mediterranean diet include the following

- whole grains
- legumes
- beans
- vegetables
- fruits
- tofu
- olives and olive oil
- herbs
- spices
- tomato sauce
- balsamic vinegar
- pesto

Foods to eat in moderation on the Mediterranean diet include the following

- seafood
- dairy
- nuts
- poultry
- honey
- seeds

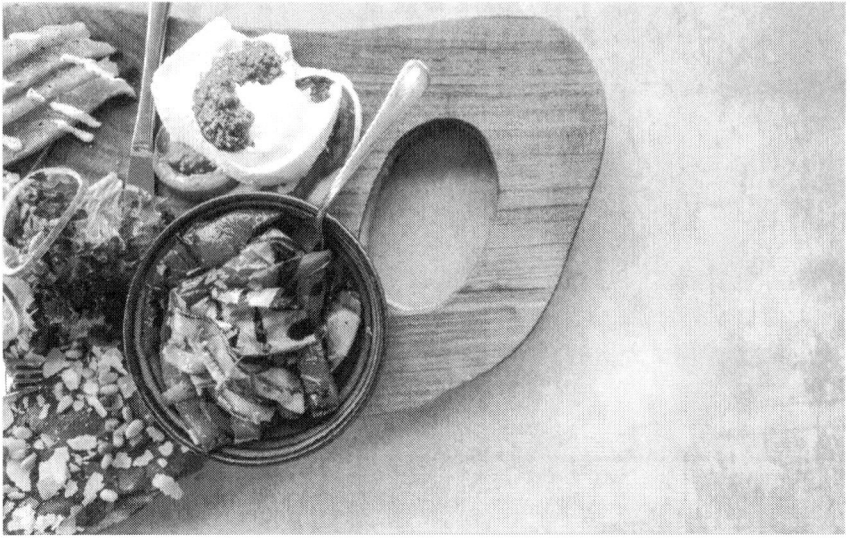

The DASH diet stands for Dietary Approaches to Stop Hypertension and is based on reducing high blood pressure, but also offers many other health benefits because it significantly reduces sodium intake and focuses on clean eating. Generally speaking, when cooking on the DASH diet, you will want to avoid adding salt to your meals in favor of other herbs and spices for flavor.

Foods to eat liberally on the DASH diet include the following

- fruits

- vegetables

- herbs and spices

- whole grains

Foods to eat in moderation on the DASH diet include the following

- seafood

- poultry

- nuts

- seeds

- beans

Foods to Eat and Foods to Avoid in an Anti-Inflammatory Diet

When starting an anti-inflammatory diet, you will want to focus on whole foods. Whole foods are foods with one ingredient, such as an apple or chicken. Foods that are high in antioxidants, such as artichokes and sweet potatoes, have anti-inflammatory properties, as do foods that are high in omega-3 fatty acids (which are a good type of fat), such as salmon and flaxseed. Here is a list of some popular foods that adhere to an anti-inflammatory diet

- ginger

- turmeric

- garlic

- flaxseed

- walnuts

- omega-3 fortified eggs and milk

- salmon

- anchovies

- sardines

- herring

- mackerel

- sweet potato

- whole grains

- broccoli

- cherries

- dark chocolate (with a minimum of 70% cocoa)

- almonds

- hazelnuts

- pecans

- kale

- collard greens

- spinach

- blueberries

- blackberries

- raspberries

- black beans

- pinto beans

- red beans

- artichokes

- apples

- avocados

- brown rice

- wild rice

- chicken breast

- turkey breast

- legumes

- seeds

- oats

- olives

- olive oil

- fermented vegetables

- yogurt

Now here are some foods that you will want to steer clear from

- processed foods

- unhealthy fats

- high-fat dairy products

- butter and margarine

- meat

- peanuts

- alcohol

- added sugars and sweeteners

- simple carbs such as white bread

Additionally, some people have sensitivities to the following foods that trigger inflammation. It is best to pay attention to your body when eating these foods to determine if your body can tolerate them. If you don't have any issues, you can include them in your diet

- gluten

- eggplant

- tomatoes

- potatoes

- peppers

- carbohydrates

Adopting a vegetarian diet is also an option for inflammation. Many people find that cutting out meat from their diet significantly reduces inflammation and makes them feel happier and healthier. Additionally, some people's bodies respond negatively to meat consumption in that they become more insulin-resistant. Because of this, you may find that getting on a vegetarian diet can help your diabetes management. However, keep in mind that cutting out meat from your diet does not give you a free pass on eating unhealthy foods or the foods mentioned above that you should try to avoid. You will still need to adhere to your anti-inflammatory diet. While chips and candy may be vegetarian, eating these types of foods while cutting out meat from your diet will not bring any change in your inflammation symptoms.

Diet for Reversal of Insulin Resistance

Whether you have diabetes or you are at risk of developing diabetes due to insulin resistance, you can make changes in your diet to target insulin resistance and help maintain your target blood sugar levels. With insulin resistance, you tend to get prolonged heightened blood sugar levels. Diets geared toward combating this issue work by lowering blood sugar levels and helping with weight loss or weight management, as being overweight is a contributing factor to insulin resistance.

When you eat foods with excessively high amounts of added sugars, your body releases a large amount of insulin to compensate. Over time, the repetition of this pattern will cause your body to become less and less sensitive to insulin. Once this happens, your blood sugar will remain high, as your cells will not be able to absorb as much of the glucose in your bloodstream. This increases your risk of developing diabetes or weakens your ability to properly manage your diabetes if you already have diabetes.

Rather than a set-in-stone diet, a diet to help reverse insulin resistance is based around you as an individual. In this case, personalization is best, as your specific needs with regard to your insulin and blood sugar levels, as well as your diabetes status, will be different from the needs of others, even if they are in a similar situation.

On a diet aimed at reversing insulin resistance, you will be eating foods like whole grains that are high in fiber, healthy fats, non-starchy vegetables, and whole foods. Here are some foods (by category) that adhere to these general guidelines:

Vegetables

- broccoli

- leafy greens

- peppers

- tomatoes

- brussels sprouts

- cauliflower

- asparagus

- green beans

- carrots

Fruits

- berries (which are also high in antioxidants)

- lemons

- limes

- oranges

- melons

- grapes

- apples

Dairy

- unsweetened yogurt

- unsweetened oat milk

- unsweetened almond milk

- low-fat cheese

Whole grains

- oats

- quinoa

- barley

- wheat

- cornmeal

- brown rice

- bulgur

- millet

- buckwheat

Legumes, nuts, and seeds

- lentils

- black beans

- kidney beans

- chickpeas

- green peas

- unsalted nuts

- seeds

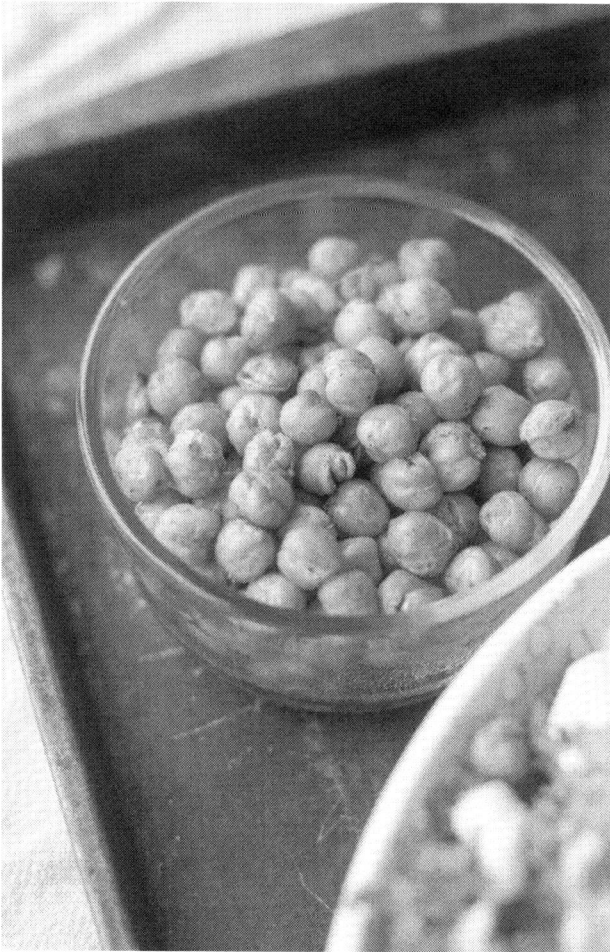

Fish

- tuna

- sardines

- salmon

- herring

- trout

- mackerel

Lean meats and meat alternatives

- skinless chicken

- skinless turkey

- tofu

- tempeh

You should also drink water as much as you can, avoiding sugary drink alternatives such as sports drinks, sodas (including diet sodas), or juices.

Additionally, here are some foods that you should try to avoid on this type of diet

- processed foods

- foods with added sugars and sugar replacements

- refined carbs

- fried foods

- unhealthy fats (saturated and trans)

Part 3:
Diabetes Management

Chapter 7:

Why Detox?

The human body is designed to naturally detox. If it was not, we would all be suffering from toxic poisoning all the time. However, there are massive amounts of synthetic chemicals circulating around that our bodies were not designed to tolerate. While the human body is quite skilled at adapting to things like this, many people are concerned about the lack of research surrounding these synthetic chemicals that are in products we use and consume on a daily basis. The idea here is that we may unintentionally be overloading our systems with toxicants, or "harmful substances which have been introduced into the environment," at a rate that our bodies cannot properly take on in its natural detoxification process (AOR Marketing, 2020).

Some examples of toxicants include "synthetic food additives, pesticides, larvicides and herbicides, heavy metals, PCBs and plasticizers, flame retardants, solvents and pharmaceutical drugs" (AOR Marketing, 2020). The good news is, we can take steps to protect our bodies from these types of potentially harmful materials.

So what is actually involved in the body's natural detox process? The focus systems and organs in the detoxification process include the following

- the cardiovascular system

- the lymphatic system

- the urinary system

- the skin

- the respiratory system

- the digestive system

- the liver

- the kidneys

- the lungs

Health Benefits of Detoxification

While the body will naturally detox, there are some steps that you can take to help the organs and systems heavily involved in the detox process stay healthy and fully functioning.

- Limit alcohol

  - Alcohol impairs your liver function. The liver is an essential organ in your body's detox process

- Prioritize sleep

  - Sleep helps restore and revitalize your brain so that it can detox

- Drink more water

  - Water helps everything in your body function a little better. It also helps the overall detox system flush out waste from your blood.

- Cut out processed foods and sugar

  - These types of foods often lead to health issues, such as diabetes, that can cause your organs to stop working as well, thus making the detox process much harder for your body.

- Eat more antioxidant-rich foods

- Antioxidants help reduce your risk of developing diseases that can negatively impact organs and systems involved in the detox process. They can also reduce any damage that free radicals (a type of harmful molecule) may have caused.

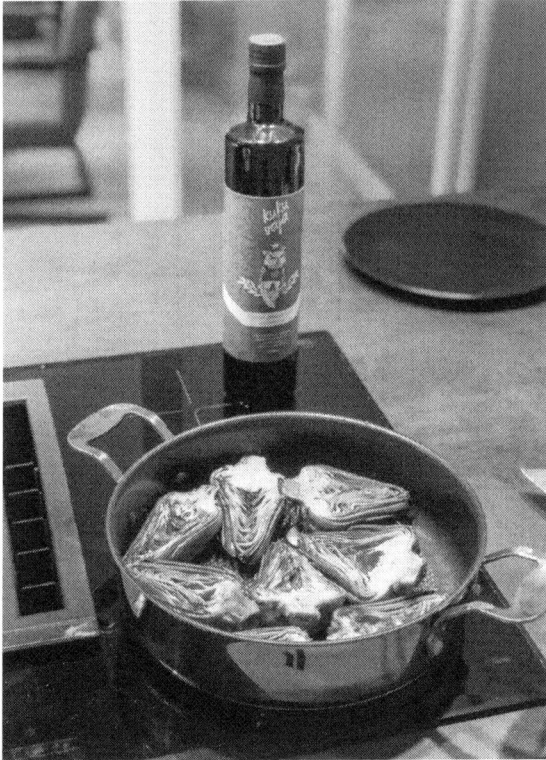

- Eat more probiotic-rich foods

  - Probiotics help aid your gut health and digestive system, which is a key system in your body's detox process and immune health.

- Cut back on salt

  - Salt intake increases water retention ("water weight"). Cutting back on salt and actually increasing your water consumption will help flush out water weight.

- Stay active
  - Staying active reduces inflammation and helps your detox system function properly.

Through these steps, you will see and feel a difference in your holistic health. This is because you are taking care of your body and the systems that are needed in the detox process. Here are some benefits you may begin to notice:

- increased energy levels

- brighter, clearer, healthier skin

- weight loss

- strengthened immune system

- less stress

- increased ability to focus and remain mentally alert

- shinier, healthier hair

- better breath

- improved mental health

- feeling lighter

- reduced inflammation

- improved sleep

- improved circulation

Those Sugars and Toxins Need to Go

Increasing your awareness of the amount of sugar that is present in the foods you regularly consume is a good place to start when cutting back on sugar intake. Make sure to read nutrition labels and pay attention to serving size. For example, you may see that your favorite snack might only have five grams of sugar when you read the nutrition label. However, upon further inspection you may see that this is per serving size, and you usually eat four times the serving size. This means that this snack actually represents twenty grams of sugar, which is already more than you should be eating in an entire day.

Cutting out sugar is one of the best ways to improve your diet and allow your body room to detox. Without all the extra sugar, your body's organs and various systems will be able to really hone in on their jobs, and as a result, leave you feeling so much better—both physically and mentally. Here are some tips on how to effectively and painlessly remove excessive amounts of sugar from your system.

- Take it slowly. Be patient and kind to yourself. Quitting sugar is not easy! But you already have the tools and the motivation within you to start. Identifying foods in your diet that have excessive amounts of added sugars is the first step. Slowly taking these foods out of your diet, rather than attempting to quit sugar cold-turkey will be easier and more sustainable. Try to eliminate added sugars from your diet over the course of two weeks, rather than overnight. Replace processed, sugary snacks with whole foods that contain natural sugar, such as fruits.

- Drink lots of water. As discussed before, dehydration can often be disguised as sugar cravings! Keeping a water bottle on hand will remind you to sip water throughout your day. Staying hydrated (with water, not sugary drinks or caffeine) will help prevent sugar cravings and help your body detox properly. If you are someone who cannot give up flavored drinks, or do not have a particular liking towards water, try adding fruit or herbs, such as cucumber and lemon slices, or mint leaves, to your water. This is a healthy and natural way to make your water more interesting and tasty.

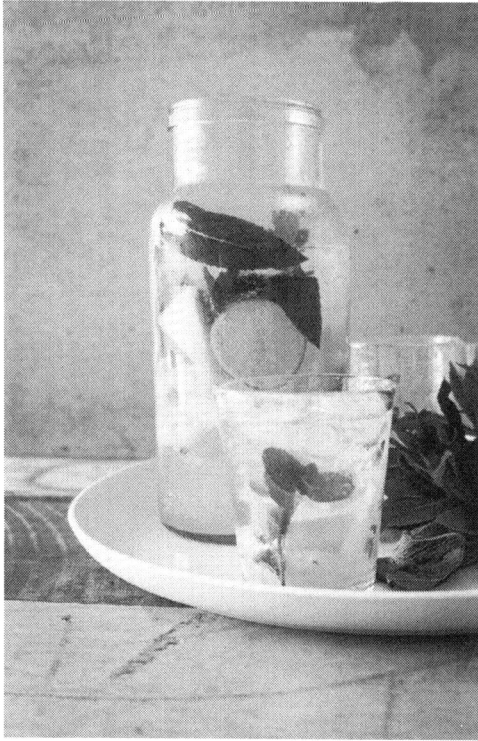

- Pay attention to your sleep patterns. When you get less than six hours of sleep, the hormones that regulate your appetite are thrown off, and because of this, you may experience increased sugar cravings. Getting proper sleep makes everything in your body function better, including detoxification.

- Reduce stress. Stress makes many people crave sugar, as sugar may seem to temporarily relieve some stress. Although recognizing that sugar does not actually help with stress in the bigger picture is a good place to start, it may be even more helpful to focus more on your stress management. Stress takes a huge toll on the body and the mind. Finding ways to deal with stress will drastically improve your holistic health. Pay attention to when you start to feel stressed out. When stress starts to manifest, try stepping outside for some fresh air, taking deep breaths, meditating, calling a close friend or family member, or any other practices that help you destress. It's important to be able to recognize what symptoms of stress look like for you, and then be able to take a moment to center yourself.

- Track your progress. Keeping a journal to write down what you are actually doing on a daily basis in terms of your sugar detox steps, as well as writing down any changes you notice in your body, will help when you want check how certain foods or the elimination of certain foods had an effect on your body. This can also help you come up with a long-term nutrition plan that is personalized for your body. Keeping a journal can also help keep you motivated to move forward. Looking back on where you started versus where you have come can be such a rewarding experience.

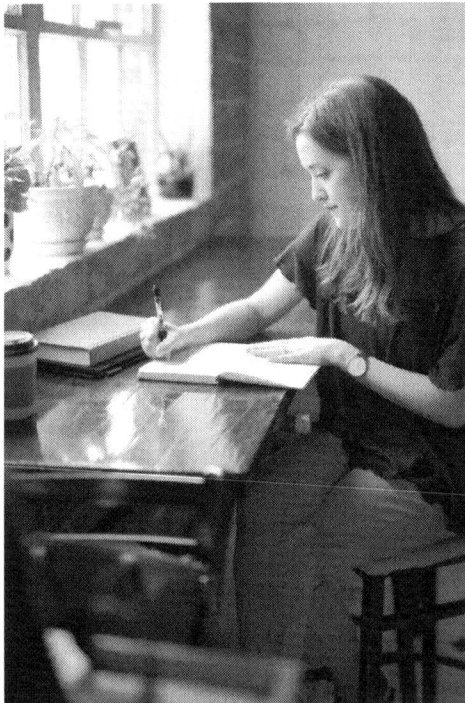

Juice Cleanse: Not Just a Trendy Word

Juice cleanses have gained mainstream popularity in recent years, as they claim to help you lose weight quickly while also detoxifying the body. On a juice cleanse, you only consume certain juices made from fruits, vegetables, and sometimes certain supplements. They advertise that by the end of the cleanse—which tends to last as little as three days to as long as three weeks—you will have lost weight, cleared up your skin, and flushed all the toxins from your body. However, they usually do not specify what kinds of toxins they are actually talking about. They also don't mention that, while only consuming fruits and vegetables for a period of time will likely cause weight loss, it can cause other health issues and will result in you gaining all of the weight back immediately once you start eating proper meals again (Devje, 2022).

When fruits and vegetables are juiced in a food processor, they lose much of their fiber. As a result, you will not feel as full from these juices as you would if you were to eat the fruit and vegetable ingredients in their whole food form, and you will not get the same amount of fiber in your diet when consuming the juice form rather than the whole food form.

That being said, there are some potential health benefits to juicing. For starters, it immediately eliminates any highly-processed foods from your diet while adding lots of vitamins and minerals from the fruit and vegetable ingredients. This is also a potentially easier way for people to start eating more fruits and vegetables. Most people do not eat nearly enough fruits and vegetables, and juicing allows for highly-concentrated amounts of fruits and vegetables. The result is you are essentially consuming many more fruits and vegetables without feeling like you are chopping up and munching on them all day.

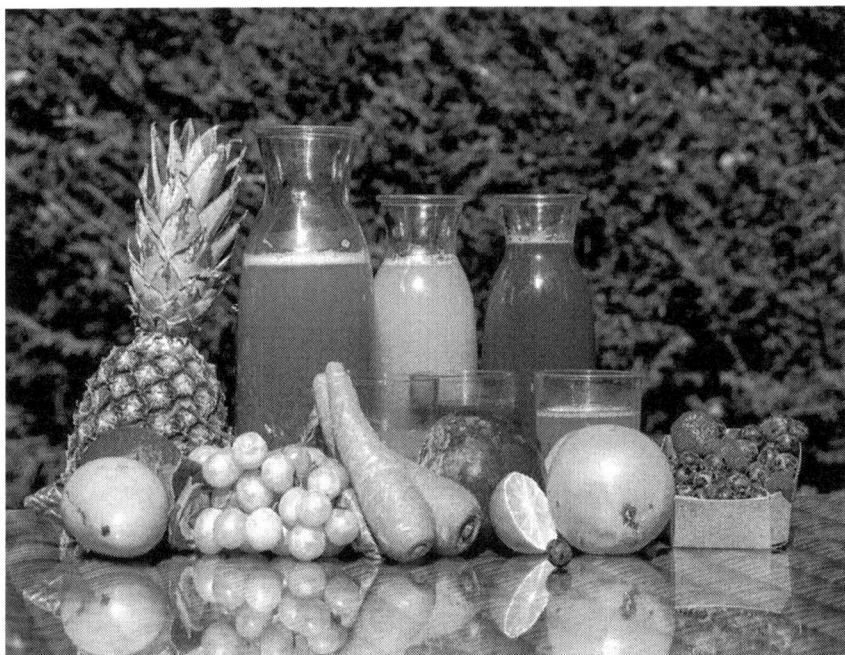

Consuming more of these kinds of foods can help increase your good gut bacteria, which, as discussed earlier, will help many aspects of your overall health. However, consuming the ingredients for these juices as whole foods provides more health benefits, including aiding your body's systems and organs in their ability to maintain detoxification functions. In the long term, you should also be eating other types of foods in addition to fruits and vegetables to maintain a balanced diet. If a juice cleanse is something that you want to try, you should speak to your doctor first.

Prediabetes Detoxification

If you are prediabetic, you will want to do everything you can to reverse your symptoms so that you are no longer at high risk for developing diabetes. Diet and exercise are the best tools that you can use to detox your system and reverse your prediabetic state.

The first step should be cutting out excess sugar and processed foods. Instead, choose proteins, healthy fats, and complex carbs. These types of foods will help keep you feeling fuller for longer, and they will also help reduce your sugar cravings. This will also help you balance your meals, and in doing so, ensure that you are getting the nutrients necessary to help your body thrive.

Stay physically active. Remaining sedentary actually leads to more sugar cravings. When you lead a more active lifestyle, you will have more energy, your insulin levels will be more easily managed, and your body will be better equipped to detox. Remember that exercise will look different for everyone. Especially when starting out, you will want to ease into an exercise routine. This can be as simple as going for a daily walk around your neighborhood. Exercise doesn't necessarily need to look like putting in hours at the gym. As long as you're moving, you are progressing!

Detoxification Recipes for Blood Sugar

Apple Cider Vinegar Detox Drink

Ingredients

- At least 8 oz. of water
- 1 tsp. cinnamon
- 1 tbsp. raw honey
- 2 tbsp. apple cider vinegar
- 2 tbsp. lemon juice

Ginger Detox Water

Ingredients

- 1-inch ginger root
- At least 8 oz. of water

Instructions

- Boil ginger root in water

- Strain into a mug

Cinnamon Detox Water

Ingredients
- 1-2 tbsp. cinnamon powder
- At least 8 oz. of water

Instructions
- Soak cinnamon in water overnight

Debunking Detox Myths

Unfortunately, in recent years, the word detox has become widely popularized and has lost its meaning. We constantly see ads for products that claim to be detoxifying. However, in reality any product can slap the word detox onto their product, regardless of whether the product has anything to do with detoxing. Detox products and diets "rarely identify the specific toxins they aim to remove or the mechanism by which they supposedly eliminate them,"(Van De Walle, 2019) and because of this, they usually do not actually do anything to help your body's natural detox process .

In reality, you cannot detox something unless it is poisoned or drugged. In other words, detox can only be accurately used when talking about a "clinical treatment of drug addiction and poisoning" (Paddock, 2009). In a sense, there really is no such thing as a detox. But the idea behind a detox is to get healthy and clear up any problem areas. The best way to do this is through good, old-fashioned diet and exercise.

The way that the word detox is marketed to consumers insinuates that the body is incapable of expelling harmful toxins on its own. However, if our bodies built up toxins without being able to get rid of them, we would all be in the hospital as we speak. Our bodies are designed to detoxify. Here are some commonly (and inaccurately) used "detox" myths.

- Myth: Your body needs detox products to help expel toxins.

  - Your body detoxes naturally, and it has multiple mechanisms for doing so. If it didn't, we would all be in serious trouble. A healthy body will be able to handle toxins just fine on its own. When your body is not able to do so, there may be a more serious issue at hand, and likely none of these popular detox products will do anything to actually help boost your body's ability to detox.

- Myth: Detoxing helps you lose weight.

  - Many detox products are also marketed to catch your eye through promises of weight loss. The idea behind this is that when the consumer believes that they can cleanse their body of toxins and lose weight at the same time, the product becomes irresistible. While it's true that this idea is incredibly appealing, the science behind it is simply inaccurate. These products or regimens may help you drop a few pounds in a short period of time, but they are not healthy or realistic to maintain in the long-term. Something like a juice cleanse may be advertised as a detoxifying weight loss regimen, but these regimens are often quite stressful for the body, especially when done without the help of a doctor. Additionally, they just don't work. As soon as the juice cleanse ends after a few days, the weight comes back. Unfortunately, if it seems too good to be true, it usually is.

- Myth: You can detox topically.

  - There are lots of topical products that are advertised as detox regimens. The idea of a topical product pulling out toxins through the pores on your skin is an appealing idea but in reality, your skin is designed to block toxins from entering the body in the first place. While you should regularly clean your skin in order to remove dirt and oil that can build up in your pores, you aren't actually removing toxins.

- Myth: You can sweat out toxins.

    o This notion is becoming increasingly popular. The idea here is that you can use exercise as a way to literally expel toxins from your body through the sweat you produce when you exercise. In reality, you do not sweat toxins—you sweat water (and a little salt). Sweating is not the body's way of expelling toxins;, it is the body's way of keeping your body temperature cool. That being said, exercise does fall in line with the general idea behind detox culture—exercise helps keep you healthy. It also helps keep your liver healthy, which is where the real detoxifying process takes place. The liver is built to detox, not our sweat glands.

The best way to keep your body healthy and "clean" is through eating a healthy diet, drinking lots of water throughout your day, and getting regular exercise. Cutting out or limiting alcohol consumption and quitting smoking if applicable will also greatly improve your overall health.

Chapter 8:

Tips for Improving Your Health

One of the very best things you can do to take charge of your health is move more. The human body was not built to sit around all day; doing so actually causes more harm than good. We need to move to stay healthy.

When we lead sedentary lifestyles, we are more likely to experience

- worsened mental health

- decreased energy levels

- poor sleep

- obesity

- diabetes or worsened management of diabetes

- heart disease

- osteoporosis

- headaches

- poor posture

- arthritis

- aches, pains, and stiffness

- increased stress

- mood swings

Adding more physical activity to your lifestyle can bring about

- strengthened immune system

- less stress

- lowered risk of heart disease

- healthy weight

- better management of blood sugar, insulin, and type 2 diabetes

- better management of blood pressure and cholesterol

- improved musculoskeletal conditions like joint and muscle stiffness and arthritis

- strengthened and denser bones

- improved kinesthesia (the body's ability to perceive movement and spatial awareness), which helps prevent falls and injury

- improved mental health

- lowered risk of bone breaking and osteoporosis

- shortened recovery time from both illness and injury

- improved sleep and daily energy levels

Keeping active throughout your day may seem like a huge challenge—especially for those who lead busier lifestyles, whether it be with a demanding job, kids, or other life factors that limit your ability to put in time at the gym. However, staying active doesn't necessarily require hours of working out every week. It is more important that you find little ways to stay active throughout your day, rather than sit around all day and then push yourself to your limit at the gym. Here are some easy ways to keep moving throughout your day:

- When driving somewhere, park farther away from your destination. Usually, we like to find the closest spot to the shop or area we are trying to get to. Actually, we often spend more time circling around the parking lot in search of a close parking spot than it would take to park a bit farther away and walk to the building.

- Take the stairs whenever possible. If you live or work a few floors up, make it a habit to take the stairs. This won't add much time (it can actually often save some time), and it won't leave you heaving for air, yet it is a good way to get into the habit of more activity.

- If you are able, choose to walk or ride a bike. Biking to work is a great way to add physical activity into your everyday routine, if this is a feasible option for you—it also helps reduce pollution and saves you gas money! If you do not live close enough to work, consider other places you frequent, such as a nearby grocery store.

- If you take public transportation, consider getting off one stop early and walking the rest of the way. This is an easy way to get outside and move, even for a relatively short amount of time.

- If the weather isn't tolerable for longer walks outside, consider going to a shopping mall or larger grocery store and walking around indoors. You will want to avoid temptations here—if you are a big spender, you might want to avoid passing by your favorite stores, or if you are walking through the aisles of a grocery store, you will want to avoid junk food aisles. However, this is a good way to get those steps in even with unfavorable weather.

- Take a walk during work breaks. It may help to get a coworker to walk with you—you can even bring your lunch and eat while you talk and walk. Depending on your work, you might often spend all of your time at your job sitting. Going outside for a break and walking around for a bit—even if it is just ten minutes—can feel invigorating, and actually help improve your work performance when you return.

- If you have someone who cleans your home or does yardwork for you, try doing it yourself for a while. This will not only help save you some money, but it will also get you moving. Household chores can actually add a lot more physical activity into your daily routine than you may realize.

- Try choosing a physical activity to do during your free time. A lot of the time, it is most tempting to just plop down on the couch at the end of the day and turn on the television. However, finding a physical activity that you enjoy just as much (or more) will help shift your perspective so that you actually want to get out and move, rather than stay seated inside. Finding other people to participate in physical activities with you can help a lot with this. For instance, instead of meeting a friend for a coffee and chat, suggest going for a walk while you chat. The more you can integrate these sorts of replacements in your daily life, the more of your day you will spend moving— likely without even feeling like you are exerting a lot of energy or "exercising." The more active your lifestyle becomes, the more exercise you will feel motivated to get and the more you will enjoy participating in increasingly physical activities.

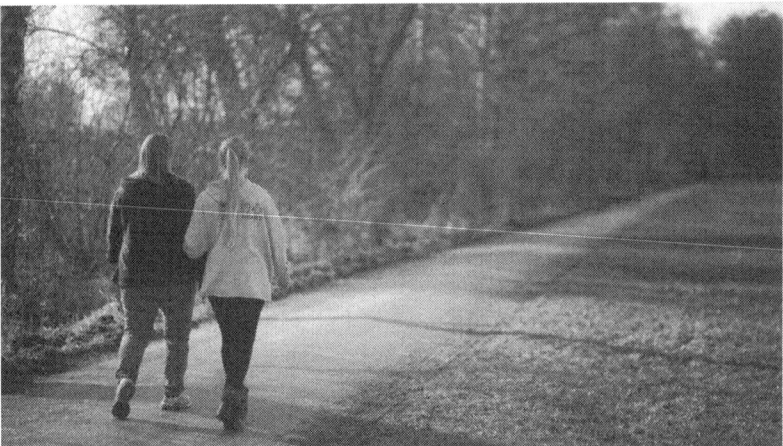

Making the Necessary Healthy Lifestyle Change

Changing your lifestyle can feel intimidating, and because of this it is best to take it slowly and focus on a few realistic goals at a time. Try writing down different, specific aspects of your life that you would like to improve. These ideas may come to you at different times. As you move through your day, try to increase your awareness of your behaviors.

For instance, maybe you catch yourself snacking on the couch while watching television and realize that this is something you do every day. Then, try to think of a small way that you can make a healthier change to this activity. For example, maybe you love watching television after a long day at work and this is not something you are willing to give up. You can work with this! Try to set a goal to only watch one or two episodes of your favorite TV show when you get home from work for the next few days. Instead of snacking while watching TV, pick up some light weights and do some basic arm exercises or do some squats during commercial breaks. This way, you are still able to enjoy watching TV while also turning into a less unhealthy "guilty pleasure."

Setting smaller goals for yourself will help you stay motivated to keep going, as you are able to more frequently rejoice in the tiny wins. Breaking up your goals into categories can also help make them more manageable. Try looking at the following categories and identifying what kinds of changes you would like to see in each (while also understanding that many of these categories will influence one another).

- nutrition

- mental health

- exercise

- water

- sleep

- diabetes management

Identifying why you want to make these changes can also make a huge impact in your motivation to change. Try taking some time to journal about what inspired you to take charge of your life, where you are currently on your journey, where you see yourself in the near future, and some specific steps that you can take to move towards that place. Remind yourself of why you are making your lifestyle changes as you work on developing your new habits.

Go For Foods With Low Glycemic Index and High Fiber

Foods with a low glycemic index (GI) are foods that have less of an effect on blood sugar. Glycemic index is measured on a scale from 0-100, zero being foods that do not affect blood sugar, and 100 being foods that have a drastic effect on blood sugar. Foods with low GI range from 1-55; foods with medium GI range from 56-69; foods with high GI range from 70-100. GI is determined by a number of different factors, such as the type of sugar that the food contains (for example, fructose versus maltose), method of preparation or cooking, starch structure, and ripeness (Coyle, 2017).

Examples of foods that score low on the GI scale include green vegetables, chickpeas, lentils, kidney beans, raw carrots, and most fruits. Examples of foods that score mid-level on the GI scale include rye bread, whole-grain bread, multigrains, raisins, pineapple, sweet corn, oat-based breakfast cereals, cherries, and bananas. Examples of foods that score high on the GI scale include potatoes, white bread, and white rice.

Carbs come in three basic forms: fiber, sugars, and starches. When you consume carbs, your body converts the starches and sugars into glucose, which then travels through your bloodstream and affects your blood sugar levels. However, your body does not absorb fiber as it passes through your body.

Benefits of eating a diet consisting of low-scoring GI foods include weight loss, lowered cholesterol, lowered blood pressure, improved diabetes management, and lowered risk of cardiovascular disease and diabetes. This is also partially due to the fact that low-GI scoring foods also tend to be higher in nutrients and fiber.

Eating foods that score low on the GI scale will help you manage your diabetes or prevent you from developing diabetes if you are prediabetic. Try swapping out foods that are high on the GI scale with foods that are low on the GI scale. These foods should also be higher in fiber. These types of foods include fruits, vegetables, beans, and grains. Swap out your white bread and white pasta for whole-grain versions of these foods.

Stress Management Skills Are Important

Stress can be a leading factor in so many health issues—both mental and physical. Many people with chronic health conditions, such as diabetes, also hold additional layers of stress related to their condition. Stress can take a physical toll on diabetes management, which adds even more stress; this can all feel like you are stuck in a never-ending cycle. The issues that stress can bring on—such as mood swings and lack of sleep—can also take an emotional toll, which can then lead to poor lifestyle choices such as remaining sedentary and eating junk food. These factors will also make diabetes management increasingly difficult. But unfortunately, many people often disregard their stress management, and put their mental health on the back burner.

Because of this, it can be beneficial to think of stress management as part of your diabetes management. Taking a holistic approach to diabetes management is much more helpful than only thinking of diabetes management in terms of blood sugar levels. So how can you take steps to improve your stress management?

- Acknowledge your stress. This can seem counterintuitive at first, but acknowledging when you are feeling stressed, rather than trying to push down or ignore the feeling, allows you to recognize triggers and then take steps to alleviate your stress. It also allows you the freedom of accepting that you are someone who experiences stress—just like every other human being. Acknowledging that stress is normal instead of feeling worse about yourself for feeling stressed will help you move past it, as opposed to entering a cycle of feeling stressed and then feeling even more stressed because you are stressed. The next time you feel stressed, take a moment, acknowledge the feeling as valid, think about what it was that made you feel this way, take a moment to breathe and center yourself, and then imagine that whatever triggered your stress is passing on by. This can help you release any negative, intrusive thoughts contributing to your feelings of stress.

- Regularly finding time to be active can also help prevent stress. Exercise releases endorphins, lowers blood pressure, helps clear your mind from lingering negative thoughts, brings you into the present, energizes you, and helps keep your body feeling good. It can also help to find an activity that you enjoy. This will help motivate you to stay active and also bring you joy! Remember that this can be as simple as taking a walk with a friend while you catch up.

- Physical relaxation activities will also bring a sense of peace. Whether it be breathing exercises, yoga, meditation, or simply taking a bath, taking time to physically decompress can make a huge difference in your mood. Practicing relaxation exercises like meditation on a regular basis can help build de-stressing activities into your daily routine. The more you are able to make a habit of these types of activities, the more well-equipped you will feel to take on the day, even when you know that you will be faced with some potentially stress-inducing challenges, such as meeting a deadline at work or having to pick up the kids from school right after a big meeting.

Keep Your ABCs In Check

If you have diabetes, it is essential to look after your ABC's, which stand for:

- A: A1C tests, which you should be getting at least twice a year, in order to measure your average blood sugar levels for the most recent 2-3 months.

- B: Blood pressure.

- C: Cholesterol levels.

- S: Stop smoking or do not take up smoking.

Your ABC goals will depend on many personal factors, such as age and any other existing conditions. However, most people with diabetes can aim for the following ABC levels:

- A1C: under 7%

- blood Pressure: under 140/90

- cholesterol LDL Levels: under 100

Managing your ABCs is so important for those with diabetes because the condition increases your risk for heart attack and stroke. On average, people with diabetes tend to have heart attacks at younger ages than the non-diabetic population. They also tend to be more deadly or more damaging than heart attacks suffered by the overall non-diabetic population. If you have diabetes, you are also at a higher risk for developing kidney disease. Regularly checking your ABCs and taking the steps to maintain your ABC goals will help prevent these life-threatening complications.

In addition to taking any medications that your doctor may put you on, you can manage your ABCs through healthy lifestyle changes. Sticking to a healthy diet that you and your doctor come up with to best suit your individual needs and goals will play a huge role in your holistic health—including your ABCs. Cutting out any smoking and also cutting out or limiting alcohol consumption as much as possible will allow you to better manage your ABCs. Exercise will also impact your ABCs, as well as your overall physical and mental health. All these steps will also allow you to either lose weight if you are overweight or maintain a healthy weight, which will lower your risk of developing other health problems including health problems that have to do with your ABCs.

Self-Care is Always Important

Many people often tend to think of self-care as an indulgence. This is because self-care is often associated with things like eating what you want, pouring yourself some wine, calling off sick from work, spending time on your hobbies, or taking a bubble bath. In reality, this doesn't actually represent what self-care truly means. While it's beneficial to do activities that relax you and make you happy, it is also essential to understand that these things must be done in balance with activities and behaviors that promote your health in the long term. This is what we mean by self-care, but this aspect of self-care is often ignored.

While it feels great to unwind at the end of the day, it is important to do so while being mindful of your health—especially when you have diabetes. If you want to eat a massive slice of cake and sit on the couch while watching a movie, this is not really self-care because it may be more harmful to you than beneficial. However, there are ways to find a happy medium between what you really want to do and what would benefit you most. For instance, choosing a healthier snack that you still enjoy while you watch a movie on the couch is a perfectly acceptable way to unwind. Practicing moderation is key here: you do not want to be sitting on the couch watching TV *all* day, nor do you want to be spiking your blood sugar with a large slice of cake. Try to find ways to unwind and take care of your health, instead of only focusing on the unwinding aspect of self-care.

Self-care also means taking all the steps discussed in this book to look after your physical and mental health and properly manage your diabetes. Think of your diabetes management as part of your overall self-care because, in reality, it is part of your overall self-care! When you take charge of your well-being, you are taking charge of your ability to manage your diabetes. It is easy for people—especially for those with diabetes who have increased stress factors—to lose motivation. However, keeping this idea of self-care and holistic health present in your mind can help keep you motivated to take better care of yourself as part of your self-care.

Don't Skip the Doctor for Checkups

Scheduling regular check-ups with your doctor should be part of your self-care routine. In doing so, you are taking essential steps to prevent other health complications and to make sure that everything is working as it should in terms of the diabetes management strategies that you and your doctor have come up with.

At your check-ups, make sure that you test your blood sugar levels with an A1C test, as well as checking your feet, eyes, blood pressure levels, kidneys, cholesterol levels, and any other issues that may be bothering you or that you want to ask your doctor about. It is beneficial to keep track of any kind of symptoms that may be bothering you or areas of your health that you notice a change in. You should also keep track of the progress that you are making with your new lifestyle changes. This way, when you go in for check-ups, you can have a list of topics to refer to when telling your doctor about changes to your health. It's common for people to schedule a doctor's appointment because a number of things are bothering them, but then once they get to their appointment, they can't think of all the symptoms they wanted to talk to their doctor about. Making a physical list as these factors arise will help you with this.

Diabetes remission refers to the state of having your blood sugar levels below the diabetic range without the help of medication in type 2 diabetes patients. Remember that this does not mean that you are "cured." Rather, it means that you are managing your type 2 diabetes symptoms well enough for your body to maintain healthy blood sugar levels on its own. Even if you are able to get to this stage, it is essential to maintain regular doctor's visits, as remission for type 2 diabetes is not set-in-stone (your blood sugar levels can still rise depending on what you eat and various other lifestyle choices and other health factors). This way, you are ensuring that everything you have been doing to get to where you are now is still working for your body (Diabetes UK, 2019).

7-Day Anti-Inflammatory Diet Plan

When starting out, it can be useful to have a meal plan in place so that you know what groceries to buy (and what not to buy) and what meals to prepare on a daily basis to ensure that you are getting balanced nutrition that adheres to your new diet. Once you get more used to the types of cooking and meals you can eat on your diet, the planning aspect will start to get a lot easier. Here is a sample week-long meal plan for an anti-inflammatory diet. Remember that before starting any diet, you should talk to your doctor to make sure that your plan will meet your individual dietary needs.

Day 1

- Breakfast: Overnight Oats

- Lunch: Spinach and Feta Frittata

- Dinner: Roasted Mediterranean Chicken, Gnocchi, and Brussels Sprouts

Day 2

- Breakfast: Green Smoothie

- Lunch: Quinoa and Citrus Salad

- Dinner: Bean Burrito

Day 3

- Breakfast: Smoked Salmon and Poached Eggs on Toast

- Lunch: Grilled Chicken and Kale Salad

- Dinner: Stuffed Sweet Potato with Hummus Dressing

Day 4

- Breakfast: Greek Yogurt with Cherries and Walnuts

- Lunch: Tuna Pita Pockets with a Side Salad

- Dinner: Chicken, Lentil, and Sweet Potato Soup

Day 5

- Breakfast: Breakfast Sandwich with a Side of Pear

- Lunch: Veggie Bowl with a Side of Orange

- Dinner: Salmon and Cauliflower Rice Bowl

Day 6

- Breakfast: Spinach and Cheese Omelet with Avocado Toast

- Lunch: Peanut, Chicken, and Zucchini Noodle Salad with a Side of Orange

- Dinner: Vegetarian Chili

Day 7

- Breakfast: Almond Butter Toast with a side of Pear

- Lunch: Mediterranean Lentil Soup with a Side of Apple

- Dinner: Kale and Avocado Salad with Edamame and Blueberries with a Side of Bread

With this meal plan, you can also have two snacks a day, between meals. Snacks can include healthy foods that align with an anti-inflammatory meal plan, such as fruits, vegetables, nuts and seeds, and plain low-fat Greek yogurt.

Anti-Inflammatory Recipes for Diabetics

Here are the ingredients and recipes for your 7-day meal plan.

Breakfast

Overnight Oats

- Ingredients

    - ½ cup rolled oats

    - 1 cup low-fat milk

    - ½ cup blueberries

    - Handful of walnuts, chopped

    - 2 tbsp. chia seeds

Green Smoothie

- Ingredients

    - 1 banana

    - ¼ avocado

    - 1 cup ice cubes

    - 1 cup unsweetened almond milk

    - 1 cup kale, chopped

    - 1 tbsp. chia seeds

    - 2 tsp. honey

Smoked Salmon and Poached Eggs on Toast

- Ingredients
    - 2 slices whole grain bread, toasted
    - ½ avocado
    - Juice from ½ lemon
    - 2 eggs, poached
    - 3.5 oz. smoked salmon
    - Handful of sliced scallions
    - 2 slices tomato
    - Black pepper

Breakfast Sandwich with a Side of Pear
- Ingredients
    - 1 egg, poached
    - Whole wheat english muffin
    - ¼ avocado
    - Handful of spinach
    - One slice tomato
    - 1 tsp. dijon mustard
    - 1 pear

Greek Yogurt with Cherries and Walnuts
- Ingredients
    - 1 cup plain low-fat Greek yogurt

- ○ Handful walnuts, chopped

- ○ ¼ cup cherries

Spinach and Cheese Omelet with Avocado Toast

- Ingredients

  - ○ For the omelet:

    - 2 eggs

    - 1 cup spinach

    - ½ oz. gruyere cheese

  - ○ For the toast:

    - ¼ avocado

    - 2 slices whole-wheat bread, toasted

    - 1 tsp. sesame seeds

Almond Butter Toast with a side of Pear

- Ingredients:

  - ○ 1 slice whole-wheat bread, toasted

  - ○ 1 tbsp. natural almond butter

  - ○ 1 pear

Lunch

Spinach and Feta Frittata

- Ingredients

  - ○ 2 eggs

- ○ 1 tsp. olive oil

- ○ ¼ onion, sliced

- ○ 1 garlic clove, grated

- ○ 1 cup spinach

- ○ ¼ cup feta cheese, crumbled

- ○ Black pepper

- Instructions

  - ○ Heat oil in a skillet or nonstick pan over medium heat.

  - ○ Cook onion until transparent. Add spinach and cook until just wilted. Transfer to a plate.

  - ○ Beat your eggs in a bowl. Add your onion and spinach to the bowl. Add your feta, and stir to combine. Season with pepper.

  - ○ Transfer egg mixture to your skillet and cook over medium heat. Cover with a lid, and continue to cook until golden and cooked through (you can check this by inserting a fork).

Quinoa and Citrus Salad

- Ingredients

  - ○ 1 cup cooked quinoa

  - ○ Slices from ½ orange

  - ○ 1 celery stalk, chopped

  - ○ Handful of Brazil nuts, chopped

- ○ ¼ cup parsley, chopped

- ○ 1 green onion, sliced

- ○ For the dressing:

    - ■ ¼ tsp. black pepper

    - ■ ¼ tsp. cinnamon

    - ■ 1 garlic clove, grated

    - ■ ½ tsp. lemon juice

    - ■ Juice from 1.5 oranges

    - ■ ½ tsp. ginger, grated

    - ■ 1 tsp. white wine vinegar

- Instructions

    - ○ Peel your oranges and set ½ orange aside. Squeeze the juice from the remaining oranges into a food processor or blender. Add the rest of the dressing ingredients to your food processor and blend until smooth.

    - ○ Cut your whole orange slices into 1-inch chunks. Transfer to a mixing bowl. Add the rest of your salad ingredients, as well as the dressing, and toss to combine.

Grilled Chicken and Kale Salad

- Ingredients

    - ○ 3 oz. chicken breast, grilled and chopped

    - ○ 3 cups kale, chopped

- ¼ cup blueberries

- Handful of unsalted almonds

- ¼ cup canned low-sodium chickpeas

- 2 tbsp. balsamic vinaigrette

Veggie Bowl with a Side of Orange
- Ingredients

  - 2 cups spinach

  - ½ cup cooked quinoa

  - ¼ cup canned low-sodium chickpeas

  - ½ cup grated carrots

  - ½ cup sugar snap peas

  - ½ cup edamame

  - 2 tbsp. carrot ginger dressing or other balsamic vinaigrette

  - 1 orange

Peanut, Chicken, and Zucchini Noodle Salad with a Side of Orange
- Ingredients

  - ¼ cup unsalted peanuts, chopped

  - 2 cups shredded chicken

  - 1 cup spiralized carrot

  - 3 cups spiralized red cabbage

  - 4 cups spiralized zucchini

- ○ ½ cup cilantro, chopped
- ○ For the dressing:
    - ■ 1 garlic clove, grated
    - ■ 1.5 tbsp. fish sauce
    - ■ 2 tbsp. low-sodium soy sauce
    - ■ ¾ cup natural peanut butter
    - ■ Juice from 1 lime
    - ■ ¾ cup hot water
    - ■ 1 tsp. hot sauce
- ○ 1 orange

Tuna Pita Pockets with a Side Salad

- ○ 3 oz. canned tuna
- ○ 1 tbsp. plain low-fat Greek yogurt
- ○ 1 tbsp. chopped red onion
- ○ 1 celery stalk, chopped
- ○ 1 sprig dill
- ○ 1 tsp. lemon juice
- ○ 6-inch whole-wheat pita
- ○ For the salad:
    - ■ 2 cups mixed greens
    - ■ Handful of cherry tomatoes, halved

- ½ cup sliced cucumbers

- 1 tbsp. lemon vinaigrette

- 1 tbsp. sunflower seeds

Mediterranean Lentil Soup (makes 6 servings; leftovers may be frozen) with a Side of Apple

- Ingredients

  - 1 cup chopped carrots

  - 3 garlic cloves, minced

  - 2 tbsp. olive oil

  - 1.5 cups chopped onion

  - 1 cup water

  - 4 cups low-sodium vegetable broth

  - 2 tsp. natural tomato paste

  - 1 can low-sodium cannellini beans

  - 1 cup lentils

  - Black pepper

  - ½ cup sun-dried tomatoes

  - 1.5 tsp. red wine vinegar

  - Handful dill, chopped

  - 1 apple

- Instructions

- Heat your oil in a large pot over medium heat. Add carrots and onions, and cook until softened (3-4 minutes).

- Add garlic and cook for 1 minute. Add tomato paste and cook for 1 minute.

- Add broth, water, lentils, tomatoes, beans, and pepper. Bring to a boil. Reduce to a simmer. Cover and cook for 30-40 minutes.

- Remove from heat, and stir in vinegar and dill.

Dinner

Bean Burrito

- Ingredients
  - ½ cup canned, low-sodium pinto beans
  - 1 tsp. cumin
  - 1 garlic clove, grated
  - ¼ cup cooked brown rice
  - ¼ cup shredded red cabbage
  - ¼ cup shredded monterey jack cheese
  - ¼ cup chopped tomatoes
  - 8-inch whole wheat tortilla
- Instructions

- Cook your beans in a pan over medium heat. Season with cumin and garlic. Continue to cook until fragrant and warmed through.

- Arrange your burrito.

Chicken, Lentil, and Sweet Potato Soup (makes 4 servings)

- Ingredients

  - 1.5 cups shredded chicken

  - 1 lb. sweet potatoes, peeled and chopped into 1-inch chunks

  - ¾ cup lentils

  - 2 tbsp. olive oil

  - 6 garlic cloves, sliced

  - 10 celery stalks, chopped

  - 1 cup spinach

  - ½ cup dill

  - 2 tbsp. lemon juice

- Instructions

  - Place lentils and potatoes in a large pot. Cover with 8 cups of water, and bring to a boil. Reduce to a simmer and cook until potatoes are tender (you can test this with a fork, 10-12 minutes).

  - Heat oil in a large skillet or nonstick pan over medium-high heat. Add garlic and celery and cook until lightly browned (12 minutes).

- Stir your garlic, celery, spinach, and chicken into the soup. Cook for 5 more minutes.

- Remove from heat and stir in lemon juice and dill.

Salmon and Cauliflower Rice Bowl (makes 2 servings)

- Ingredients

    - 2 salmon filets

    - 1 dozen brussels sprouts, halved

    - 1 bunch kale, chopped

    - 1 head cauliflower, minced into cauliflower rice in a food processor

    - 1 tsp. curry powder

    - 3 tbsp. coconut or olive oil

    - For the salmon marinade:

        - 1 tsp. dijon mustard

        - 1 tsp. sesame oil

        - 1 tbsp. sesame seeds

        - ¼ cup tamari sauce

- Instructions

    - Preheat your oven to 350°F.

    - Line a baking sheet with foil and add your brussels sprouts. Drizzle with 1 tbsp. oil. Place in the oven and roast for 20 minutes.

    - Whisk your marinade ingredients together in a bowl.

- Remove brussels sprouts from the oven and add salmon to the baking sheet. Drizzle the salmon with your marinade. Place the baking sheet in the oven and roast for 15 more minutes.

- Heat 1 tbsp. oil in a pan over medium-high heat. Add your kale and cook until wilted (2-3 minutes). Transfer kale to a plate.

- Heat 1 tbsp. oil in a pan over medium-high heat. Add your cauliflower rice, and season with curry powder. Cook for 2-3 more minutes.

- Remove the baking sheet from the oven. Divide your cauliflower and kale portions between two bowls. Divide salmon and brussels sprouts portions between two bowls.

Stuffed Sweet Potato with Hummus Dressing

- Ingredients

  - 1 sweet potato

  - ¾ cup kale, chopped

  - 1 cup canned low-sodium black beans

  - ¼ cup hummus

- Instructions

  - Puncture your sweet potato all over with a fork. Microwave 7-10 minutes.

  - Cook your kale in a pan over medium-high heat until wilted. Add beans and 1-2 tbsp. water if needed. Cook for 1-2 more minutes.

- Open the sweet potato and stuff with kale and beans.

- Drizzle with hummus.

Kale and Avocado Salad with Edamame and Blueberries with a Side of Bread (makes 4 servings)

- Ingredients

  - 1 avocado, chopped

  - 1 cup blueberries

  - 6 cups kale, chopped

  - 1 cup edamame

  - ½ cup goat cheese, crumbled

  - ¼ cup unsalted almonds, sliced

  - 1 cup cherry tomatoes, halved

  - For the dressing:

    - ¼ cup olive oil

    - Juice from ½ lemon

    - 1 tbsp. chives, minced

    - 1 tsp. dijon mustard

  - 1 slice whole-wheat baguette

Roasted Mediterranean Chicken, Gnocchi, and Brussels Sprouts (makes 4 servings)

- Ingredients

  - 1 lb. brussels sprouts, halved

- 4 boneless, skinless chicken thighs

- 16 oz. gnocchi

- ½ red onion, sliced

- 1 cup cherry tomatoes, halved

- 1 tbsp. red wine vinegar

- 4 tbsp. olive oil

- Black pepper

- 2 garlic cloves, minced

- 2 tbsp. oregano

- Instructions

  - Preheat your oven to 450°F.

  - Combine 2 tbsp. Oil, 1 tbsp. oregano, 1 garlic clove, and some black pepper in a large bowl. Add your onion, gnocchi, and brussels sprouts and toss. Add chicken and toss. Remove chicken and set aside.

  - Line a large baking sheet. Transfer your brussels sprouts mixture to the baking sheet, spreading it out evenly. Nestle in your chicken thighs. Roast for 10 minutes.

  - Remove the baking sheet from the oven and mix in your tomatoes. Transfer back to the oven and cook for 10 more minutes.

  - Remove from the oven and drizzle with vinegar and the rest of your oil.

Vegetarian Chili (makes 4 servings)

- Ingredients

    - 2 carrots, chopped

    - 1 bell pepper, chopped

    - 1 red onion, chopped

    - 2 celery stalks, chopped

    - 2 tbsp. olive oil

    - 4 garlic cloves, minced

    - 1 can pinto beans

    - 2 cans black beans

    - 2 cans tomatoes, diced

    - 2 cups water or low-sodium vegetable broth

    - 2 tbsp. chili powder

    - 2 tsp. cumin

    - 1.5 tsp. paprika

    - 1 tsp. oregano

    - 1 bay leaf

    - 2 tbsp. cilantro, chopped

    - 2 tsp. red wine vinegar

    - Avocado, sliced

    - Cheddar cheese, grated

- Instructions

  - Heat your oil in a large pot over medium. Add your onion, carrot, celery, and bell pepper. Cook until the onion becomes translucent (7-10 minutes).

  - Add chili powder, garlic, paprika, cumin, and oregano. Cook for 1 more minute.

  - Add tomatoes, beans, broth, and bay leaf. Bring to a simmer and cook for 30 minutes.

  - Remove from heat and discard bay leaf. Mash your chili with a potato masher so that it thickens a bit. Mix in your cilantro and vinegar. Divide among 4 bowls and top with your garnishes.

Conclusion

Sugar addiction is an epidemic that's sweeping the population—and it's only getting worse. The risk factors and complications of diabetes in combination with sugar addiction are too dangerous to ignore, which is why you have already taken the first step in making a change. The truth is, sugar is in nearly every prepared food out there, and what's worse is it's intentionally being put in our food to keep us coming back. By actively changing your diet to include more whole foods, you are fighting against this dangerous system.

Learning more about your body and all its mechanisms allows you to develop the tools needed to take your health into your own hands. Natural healing from food is an effective way to reverse unfavorable symptoms—including certain diabetes symptoms—that your current diet may be causing. Now that you have all the tools to move forward in your holistic journey, go out there and use them!

If you enjoyed this book, please leave a review!

Author Bio

Laura Garrett was born and raised in a small town in the American Midwest where she developed a love for cooking at a young age. Her mother was an excellent cook, and Laura often spent time in the kitchen with her, learning cooking and baking basics. As she grew older, Laura became more and more interested in trying out new recipes and experimenting with different flavors and ingredients. After completing high school, Laura decided to pursue her passion for cooking by enrolling in culinary school. She excelled in her studies and upon graduation, landed a job as a line cook at a popular restaurant. Over the years, Laura worked her way up the ranks and eventually became the head chef at the restaurant.

In her spare time, Laura enjoys sharing her love for cooking with others by hosting dinner parties and cooking classes. It was at one of these dinner parties that she met her future husband, a food critic who encouraged her to turn her passion for cooking into a career.

Laura took his advice and began working on a cookbook for beginners. She wanted to create a resource for people who were just starting out in the kitchen, and wanted to make it as approachable and user-friendly as possible. After countless hours of testing and refining recipes, Laura's cookbook was finally published. The cookbook was a hit, and Laura quickly gained a loyal following of home cooks who appreciated her easy-to-follow recipes and friendly, approachable style. Laura followed up the success of her first cookbook with several more—each one focusing on a different aspect of cooking, such as healthy eating, vegetarian cooking, and baking.

As her career continued to grow, Laura began exploring other interests beyond the kitchen. She had always been a creative person, and she discovered a love for crafting and DIY projects. She started a blog to document her projects and share her knowledge with others, and it wasn't long before she was approached by a publisher to write a book on the subject.

Laura's hobby book was a hit, and she followed it up with several more, covering a wide range of topics such as gardening, knitting, and home decor. She found that she enjoyed the creative process of writing about her hobbies just as much as she enjoyed cooking, so she began to split her time between the two pursuits.

Today, Laura is a successful cookbook and hobby book author, known for her ability to make even the most complex tasks approachable and enjoyable for beginners. She continues to inspire and educate people through her work, sharing her love of cooking and hobbies with a wider audience.

References

23 Nutrition Therapy Team. (2020, December 4). *How to heal SIBO: The 3 types*. 23 Nutrition Therapy. https://www.23nutritiontherapy.com/how-to-heal-sibo-the-3-types/

AANMC. (2019, November 7). *Naturopathic approaches to gut health*. AANMC. https://aanmc.org/naturopathic-news/naturopathic-approaches-to-gut-health/#:~:text=The%20naturopathic%20approach%20for%20treatment

Ahmed, A. (2002, April 1). History of diabetes mellitus. Saudi medical journal, *23*(4), 373-8. https://pubmed.ncbi.nlm.nih.gov/11953758/

Algera, J., Colomier, E., & Simrén, M. (2019). The dietary management of patients with irritable bowel syndrome: A narrative review of the existing and emerging evidence. *Nutrients*, *11*(9), 2162. https://doi.org/10.3390/nu11092162

American Diabetes Association. (n.d.). *Know your ABC's of diabetes!* KYD Diabetes https://www.kydiabetes.net/siteadmin/ui/kdn_theme/pdf/Know%20Your%20ABCs%20of%20Diabetes.pdf

Anthony, K. (2018, August 16). *SIBO diet 101: What you should and shouldn't eat*. Healthline. https://www.healthline.com/health/sibo-diet

AOR Marketing. (2020, June 15). *Detoxification organs – What are they and what do they do?* Advanced Orthomolecular Research. https://aor.ca/detoxification-organs-what-are-they-and-what-do-they-do/#:~:text=The%20liver%20is%20the%20primary

Are cravings caused by a hormonal imbalance? (Hint: Yes!). (n.d.). *The Riegal Center.* https://www.theriegelcenter.com/blog/are-cravings-caused-by-a-hormonal-imbalance-hint-yes

Arora, S. (2013, November 1). *How to stop sugar cravings.* Women's Health Network. https://www.womenshealthnetwork.com/blood-sugar/sugar-cravings/

Fact or fiction: Making sense of detox myths. (2021, December 21). Ask the Scientists. https://askthescientists.com/detox-myths/

Asp, K. (2022, November 30). *8 everyday ways to improve your gut health naturally.* Real Simple. https://www.realsimple.com/how-to-improve-gut-health-naturally-6833619

Atoyebi, D. (n.d.). *Signs of poor gut health.* Piedmont. https://www.piedmont.org/living-better/signs-of-poor-gut-health

Avena, N. M., Rada, P., & Hoebel, B. G. (2008). Evidence for sugar addiction: Behavioral and neurochemical effects of intermittent, excessive sugar intake. *Neuroscience & Biobehavioral Reviews, 32*(1), 20–39. https://doi.org/10.1016/j.neubiorev.2007.04.019

Bachus, T. (2018, May 4). *8 steps to a healthier microbiome.* Clean Eating. https://www.cleaneatingmag.com/clean-diet/8-steps-to-a-healthier-microbiome/

Ball, J. (2019, September). *Sheet-pan chicken thighs with brussels sprouts & gnocchi.* Eating Well. https://www.eatingwell.com/recipe/276146/sheet-pan-chicken-thighs-with-brussels-sprouts-gnocchi/https://www.icliniq.com/articles/alternative-medicine/detoxification?amp=1

Banu, D. (2019, February 22). *Detoxification - Ways to detoxify your body.* Icliniq. https://www.icliniq.com/articles/alternative-medicine/detoxification?amp=1

Behring, S. (2021, July 28). *Type 4 diabetes: Causes, symptoms, risk factors, and more.* Healthline. https://www.healthline.com/health/diabetes/type-4-diabetes

Berzin, R. (2018, August 8). *Why sugar makes you feel bad and how to detox.* Parsley Health. https://www.parsleyhealth.com/blog/how-to-detox-from-sugar/

Bi-phasic diet for SIBO: The ultimate guide. (2022b, April 11). Essential Stacks. https://essentialstacks.com/blogs/gut-health/bi-phasic-diet-sibo

Bolen, B. (2023, January 3). *What to eat when you have SIBO.* Verywell Health. https://www.verywellhealth.com/the-elemental-diet-for-sibo-and-ibs-1945000

Boulangé, C. L., Neves, A. L., Chilloux, J., Nicholson, J. K., & Dumas, M.-E. (2016). Impact of the gut microbiota on inflammation, obesity, and metabolic disease. *Genome Medicine, 8*(1). https://doi.org/10.1186/s13073-016-0303-2

Boyers, L. (2014, July 17). *Telltale signs your gut is out of whack, plus what to do about it.* Mind Body Green. https://www.mindbodygreen.com/articles/signs-of-an-unhealthy-gut

Brody, B. (2017, January 24). *Anti-inflammatory diet: Road to good health?* Web MD. https://www.webmd.com/diet/anti-inflammatory-diet-road-to-good-health

Brown, M. J. (2017, November 12). *Does sugar cause inflammation in the body?* Healthline. https://www.healthline.com/nutrition/sugar-and-inflammation

Brutsaert, E. (2022a, September). *Complications of diabetes mellitus - Endocrine and metabolic disorders.* MSD Manuals. https://www.msdmanuals.com/professional/endocrine-and-metabolic-disorders/diabetes-mellitus-and-disorders-of-carbohydrate-metabolism/complications-of-diabetes-mellitus

Brutsaert, E. (2022b, October). *Diabetes mellitus (DM)*. MSD Manuals. https://www.msdmanuals.com/home/hormonal-and-metabolic-disorders/diabetes-mellitus-dm-and-disorders-of-blood-sugar-metabolism/diabetes-mellitus-dm

Bull, M. J., & Plummer, N. T. (2014). Part 1: The human gut microbiome in health and disease. *Integrative Medicine (Encinitas, Calif.)*, *13*(6), 17–22. https://www.ncbi.nlm.nih.gov/pmc/articles/PMC4566439/

Burkhart, A. (2021, May 30). *SIBO diet: Which diet is best for SIBO?* The Celiac MD. https://theceliacmd.com/the-sibo-diet/#:~:text=The%20elemental%20diet%20formula%20is

The brain-gut connection. (2019). Hopkins Medicine. https://www.hopkinsmedicine.org/health/wellness-and-prevention/the-brain-gut-connection

The causes and effects of inflammation.(2020, April 30). El Camino Health. https://www.elcaminohealth.org/stay-healthy/blog/causes-effects-of-inflammation#:~:text=Over%20time%2C%20chronic%20inflammation%20can

CDC. (2018, August 6). *Diabetes mental health*. Centers for Disease Control and Prevention. https://www.cdc.gov/diabetes/managing/mental-health.html

CDC. (2019). *Diabetes and your feet*. Centers for Disease Control and Prevention. https://www.cdc.gov/diabetes/library/features/healthy-feet.html

CDC. (2020, September 23). *Diabetes and nerve damage*. Centers for Disease Control and Prevention. https://www.cdc.gov/diabetes/library/features/diabetes-nerve-damage.html

CDC. (2021a). *Diabetes and your heart*. Centers for Disease Control and Prevention.

https://www.cdc.gov/diabetes/library/features/diabetes-and-heart.html

CDC. (2021b, May 7). *Diabetes and chronic kidney disease.* Centers for Disease Control and Prevention. https://www.cdc.gov/diabetes/managing/diabetes-kidney-disease.html

CDC. (2021c, May 7). *Diabetes and oral health.* Centers for Disease Control and Prevention. https://www.cdc.gov/diabetes/managing/diabetes-oral-health.html

CDC. (2021d, October 13). *Diabetes and hearing loss.* Centers for Disease Control and Prevention. https://www.cdc.gov/diabetes/managing/diabetes-hearing-loss.html

CDC. (2022a, March 9). *Prevent diabetes complications.* Centers for Disease Control and Prevention. https://www.cdc.gov/diabetes/managing/problems.html#:~:t ext=Common%20diabetes%20health%20complications%20inc lude

CDC. (2022b, April 5). *Diabetes risk factors.* Centers for Disease Control and Prevention. https://www.cdc.gov/diabetes/basics/risk-factors.html#:~:text=Are%2045%20years%20or%20older

CDC. (2022c, June 3). *About adult BMI.* Centers for Disease Control and Prevention. https://www.cdc.gov/healthyweight/assessing/bmi/adult_bmi /index.html

CDC. (2022d, December 14). *Steps to help you stay healthy with diabetes.* Centers for Disease Control and Prevention. https://www.cdc.gov/diabetes/library/4steps.html#:~:text=S TEP%202%3A%20Know%20your%20diabetes

Center for Healthy Eating and Activity Research. (2021, April 13). *10 ways to make lifestyle changes easy.* CHEAR.

https://chear.ucsd.edu/blog/10-ways-to-make-lifestyle-changes-easy

Chan, S. L. (2020, January 1). *Chapter ten - Microbiome and cancer treatment: Are we ready to apply in clinics?* (J. Sun, Ed.). ScienceDirect; Academic Press. https://www.sciencedirect.com/science/article/abs/pii/S1877 11732030048X

Chen, L., Chen, R., Wang, H., & Liang, F. (2015, May 28). *Mechanisms linking inflammation to insulin resistance.* Hindawi. https://www.hindawi.com/journals/ije/2015/508409/

Cimperman, S. (2016, January 11). *Detoxification for prediabetes.* Naturopathic Doctor News and Review. https://ndnr.com/detoxification-medicine/detoxification-for-prediabetes/

Cleveland Clinic. (2021, March 28). *Diabetes mellitus: An overview.* Cleveland Clinic. https://my.clevelandclinic.org/health/diseases/7104-diabetes-mellitus-an-overview

Cleveland Clinic. (2022a, February 2). *Anti-inflammatory diet: What to eat (and avoid).* Cleveland Clinic. https://health.clevelandclinic.org/anti-inflammatory-diet/amp/

Cleveland Clinic. (2022b, June 9). *How your gut microbiome impacts your health.* Cleveland Clinic. https://health.clevelandclinic.org/gut-microbiome/amp/

Collins, K. (2021, August 31). *DASH diet vs Mediterranean diet: Is one a better choice?* Karen Collins Nutrition. https://karencollinsnutrition.com/dash-diet-vs-mediterranean-diet-is-one-a-better-choice/

Complications of diabetes. (2022a). Diabetes UK. https://www.diabetes.org.uk/Guide-to-diabetes/Complications

Corleone, J. (2022, September 28). *7-day anti-inflammatory meal plan & recipe prep*. Verywell Fit. https://www.verywellfit.com/7-day-anti-inflammatory-meal-plan-and-recipe-prep-6740018

Coyle, D. (2017). *A beginner's guide to the low-glycemic diet*. Healthline. https://www.healthline.com/nutrition/low-glycemic-diet

Cresci, G. A. M., & Izzo, K. (2019, January 1). *Chapter 4 - Gut microbiome*. ScienceDirect. https://www.sciencedirect.com/science/article/pii/B9780128143308000044

Crichton-Stuart, C. (2022, March 10). *Anti-inflammatory diet meal plan: 26 healthful recipes*. Medical News Today. https://www.medicalnewstoday.com/articles/322897

Cumbers, J. (2021, February 17). *America, your diet is killing you: Why the glucose crisis will be worse than the opioid crisis*. Forbes. https://www.forbes.com/sites/johncumbers/2021/02/17/america-your-diet-is-killing-you-why-the-glucose-crisis-will-be-worse-than-the-opioid-crisis/amp/

Cunha, J. P. (2019, July 18). *Low FODMAP diet for IBS: List of foods to eat and avoid*. Medicine Net. https://www.medicinenet.com/low_fodmap_diet_list_of_foods_to_eat_and_avoid/article.htm

Dalkin, G. (2019, March). *Really green smoothie*. Eating Well. https://www.eatingwell.com/recipe/270514/really-green-smoothie/

Dandona, P. (2004). Inflammation: the link between insulin resistance, obesity and diabetes. *Trends in immunology*, *25*(1), 4–7. https://doi.org/10.1016/j.it.2003.10.013

Dansinger, M. (2016, October 31). *What are ketones and their tests?* Web MD. https://www.webmd.com/diabetes/ketones-and-their-tests

Dansinger, M. (2021, February 7). *Managing stress when you have diabetes*. WebMD. https://www.webmd.com/diabetes/managing-stress

Davis, N. (2017, August 25). *Is sugar really as addictive as cocaine? Scientists row over effect on body and brain.* The Guardian. https://amp.theguardian.com/society/2017/aug/25/is-sugar-really-as-addictive-as-cocaine-scientists-row-over-effect-on-body-and-brain

Davis, T. (n.d.). *SIBO diets: diet plans and food lists.* The Berkeley Well-Being Institute. Retrieved January 18, 2023, from https://www.berkeleywellbeing.com/sibo-diet.html

Detoxing the body: 9 incredible health benefits of a great detox program. (2017, October 5). My Vita Wellness Institute. https://www.myvitawellness.com/9-health-benefits-detoxing-the-body/

Detrano, J. (n.d.). *Sugar addiction: more serious than you think.* Rutgers. https://alcoholstudies.rutgers.edu/sugar-addiction-more-serious-than-you-think

Devje, S. (2022, February 7). *Should you try a juice cleanse? Benefits, downsides, safety.* Healthline. https://www.healthline.com/nutrition/juice-cleanse

Diabetes - Are you at risk? (2022a, November 15). Health Hub. https://www.healthhub.sg/live-healthy/1128/diabetes-are-you-at-risk

Diabetes management and stress. (2022b, November 15). Health Hub.https://www.healthhub.sg/live-healthy/1440/diabetes-and-stress-problems

Diabetes myths and facts Information. (n.d.). Mount Sinai. https://www.mountsinai.org/health-library/special-topic/diabetes-myths-and-facts

Diabetes remission. (2019). Diabetes UK. https://www.diabetes.org.uk/guide-to-diabetes/managing-your-diabetes/treating-your-diabetes/type2-diabetes-remission

Eckelkamp, S. (2021, January 10). *SIBO treatment: How to treat SIBO and prevent recurrence.* Parsley Health. https://www.parsleyhealth.com/blog/sibo-treatment/

Elite Medical Center. (2021, January 2). *6 ways to remove sugar from your diet.* Elite Medical Center. https://elitelv.com/6-ways-to-remove-sugar-from-your-diet/amp/

Escobar, S.-N. (2021, February 6). *5 surprising causes of menopause sugar cravings.* Menopause Better. https://menopausebetter.com/5-surprising-ways-to-cut-sugar-cravings/

Espina, R. (2022, November 9). *Health benefits of probiotics for gut health.* Longevity Technology. https://longevity.technology/lifestyle/health-benefits-of-probiotics-for-gut-health/

Feiereisen, S. (2022, October 26). *7 ways to break a sugar addiction and curb cravings for good.* Real Simple. https://www.realsimple.com/health/nutrition-diet/healthy-eating/how-to-break-sugar-addiction

Felman, A. (2019, March 27). *Diet and insulin resistance: Foods to eat and diet tips.* Medical News Today. https://www.medicalnewstoday.com/articles/316569

Felman, A. (2022, April 14). *Insulin resistance diet: What to eat and why it's personal.* Join Zoe. https://joinzoe.com/learn/insulin-resistance-diet.amp

Fields, H. (2014). *The gut: where bacteria and immune system meet.* Hopkinsmedicine.org. https://www.hopkinsmedicine.org/research/advancements-in-research/fundamentals/in-depth/the-gut-where-bacteria-and-immune-system-meet

Filipovic, J. (2013, September 26). *The way America eats is killing us. Something has to change.* The Guardian. https://amp.theguardian.com/commentisfree/2013/sep/26/american-diet-report-card-unhealty

5 SIBO diets compared - SCD vs biphasic vs Cedars Sinai & 2 more. (2022a, April 5). Essential Stacks. https://essentialstacks.com/blogs/gut-health/sibo-diets-compared#12

Fletcher, J. (2022, December 23). *Anti-inflammatory diet: Food list and tips.* Medical News Today. https://www.medicalnewstoday.com/articles/320233

FODMAP food list. (2022, September 1). IBS Diets.https://www.ibsdiets.org/fodmap-diet/fodmap-food-list/

Foolproof spinach and feta frittata. (n.d.). Healthy Mummy. https://www.healthymummy.com/recipe/foolproof-spinach-feta-frittata/

Ford, K. (2011, July 8). *Low glycemic and high fiber foods.* Healthfully. https://healthfully.com/257598-low-glycemic-and-high-fiber-foods.html

The 4 R's of gut health. (n.d.). The Nutritional Institute.https://thenutritionalinstitute.com/resources/blog/292-the-4-r-s-of-gut-health

14 simple ways to convert your sedentary lifestyle. (2011, March 15). Business Insider. https://www.businessinsider.com/14-simple-ways-to-convert-your-sedentary-lifestyle-2011-4?amp

Furman, D., Campisi, J., Verdin, E., Carrera-Bastos, P., Targ, S., Franceschi, C., Ferrucci, L., Gilroy, D. W., Fasano, A., Miller, G. W., Miller, A. H., Mantovani, A., Weyand, C. M., Barzilai, N., Goronzy, J. J., Rando, T. A., Effros, R. B., Lucia, A., Kleinstreuer, N., & Slavich, G. M. (2019). Chronic inflammation in the etiology of disease across the life span. *Nature Medicine, 25*(12), 1822–1832. https://doi.org/10.1038/s41591-019-0675-0

Gérard, C., & Vidal, H. (2019). Impact of gut microbiota on host glycemic control. *Frontiers in Endocrinology, 10.* https://doi.org/10.3389/fendo.2019.00029

Ghyselinck, J., Verstrepen, L., Moens, F., Van Den Abbeele, P., Bruggeman, A., Said, J., Smith, B., Barker, L. A., Jordan, C., Leta, V., Chaudhuri, K. R., Basit, A. W., & Gaisford, S. (2021). Influence of probiotic bacteria on gut microbiota composition and gut wall function in an in-vitro model in patients with Parkinson's disease. *International journal of pharmaceutics: X, 3,* 100087. https://doi.org/10.1016/j.ijpx.2021.100087

Gibson, B. (2022, May 17). *Here's why you're craving sugar all the time—Plus tips on how to stop.* Real Simple. https://www.realsimple.com/health/nutrition-diet/healthy-eating/why-am-i-craving-sugar

Grant, L. (2020). *Kale & avocado salad with blueberries & edamame.* Eating Well. https://www.eatingwell.com/recipe/280172/kale-avocado-salad-with-blueberries-edamame/

Green, J. (2022, October 31). *5 common myths about type 2 diabetes.* Duke Health. https://www.dukehealth.org/blog/5-common-myths-about-type-2-diabetes

Gunnars, K. (2018, November 13). *Probiotics 101: A simple beginner's guide.* Healthline. https://www.healthline.com/nutrition/probiotics-101

Harer, K. (2021, March 8). *IBS diet: What to do and what to avoid.* About IBS. https://aboutibs.org/treatment/ibs-diet/ibs-diet-what-to-do-and-what-to-avoid/

Harvard Health Publishing. (2013, July 1). *How to break the sugar habit-and help your health in the process.* Harvard Health. https://www.health.harvard.edu/staying-healthy/how-to-break-the-sugar-habit-and-help-your-health-in-the-process

Harvard Health Publishing. (2017, May). *The sweet danger of sugar.* Harvard Health. https://www.health.harvard.edu/heart-health/the-sweet-danger-of-sugar#:~:text=Over%20time%2C%20this%20can%20lead

Harvard School of Public Health. (2017, August 16). *The microbiome.* HSPH. https://www.hsph.harvard.edu/nutritionsource/microbiome/#:~:text=The%20microbiome%20consists%20of%20microbes

Higuera, V. (2020, June 5). *How to reverse prediabetes naturally: 8 tips to try now.* Healthline. https://www.healthline.com/health/diabetes/how-to-reverse-prediabetes-naturally

Ho, V. (2014, November 7). *How gut bacteria affects your food cravings.* Gut Dr. https://gutdr.com/how-gut-bacteria-affects-food-cravings/#:~:text=Scientists%20have%20largely%20debunked%20the

Howard, J. (2020, July). *Peanut zucchini noodle salad with chicken.* Eating Well. https://www.eatingwell.com/recipe/280559/peanut-zucchini-noodle-salad-with-chicken/

Huizen, J. (2020, December 24). *How gut microbes contribute to good sleep.* Medical News Today. https://www.medicalnewstoday.com/articles/how-gut-microbes-contribute-to-good-sleep

Illiades, C. (2020, August 10). *Diet do's and don'ts for IBS.* Health Grades. https://www.healthgrades.com/right-care/irritable-bowel-syndrome/diet-dos-and-donts-for-ibs

Illiano, P., Brambilla, R., & Parolini, C. (2020). The mutual interplay of gut microbiota, diet and human disease. *The FEBS Journal,* *287*(5), 833–855. https://doi.org/10.1111/febs.15217

Iron Orr Fitness. (2022, January 2). *Trendy cleanses and other things, do they really work?* Iron Orr Fitness. https://ironorrfitness.com/trendy-cleanses-and-other-things-do-they-really-work/

Is sugar more addictive than cocaine? (2017, September 20). New Hall Hospital. https://www.newhallhospital.co.uk/news/is-sugar-more-addictive-than-cocaine#:~:text=Drug%2Dlike%20effects&text=The%20research%20scientists%20claim%20that

Jabr, F. (2013, July 15). *Is sugar really toxic? Sifting through the evidence.* Scientific American. https://blogs.scientificamerican.com/brainwaves/is-sugar-really-toxic-sifting-through-the-evidence/

Jacques, A., Chaaya, N., Beecher, K., Ali, S. A., Belmer, A., & Bartlett, S. (2019). The impact of sugar consumption on stress driven, emotional and addictive behaviors. *Neuroscience & Biobehavioral Reviews, 103,* 178–199. https://doi.org/10.1016/j.neubiorev.2019.05.021

Karmakar, S. (2022, August 23). *High blood sugar: 5 healthy detox drinks to keep diabetes under control.* The Health Site. https://www.thehealthsite.com/fitness/diet/high-blood-sugar-5-healthy-detox-drink-recipes-to-keep-diabetes-under-control-902977/amp/

Kennedy, M., & Rifkin, M. (2021, December 14). *SIBO diet: Best foods to eat and which to avoid.* Insider. https://www.insider.com/guides/health/diet-nutrition/sibo-diet?amp

Khatri, M. (2022, February 15). *Learn about diabetes complications.* Web MD. https://www.webmd.com/diabetes/diabetes-complications

Kho, Z. Y., & Lal, S. K. (2018, August 14). *The human gut microbiome – A potential controller of wellness and disease.* Frontiers. https://www.frontiersin.org/articles/10.3389/fmicb.2018.01835/full

Killing Thyme. (2017, January 15). *Smoked salmon + poached eggs on toast.* Killing Thyme.

https://www.killingthyme.net/2017/01/15/smoked-salmon-poached-eggs-on-toast/

King, H. *Hippocrates Now*. Bloomsbury Collections. https://www.bloomsburycollections.com/book/hippocrates-now-the-father-of-medicine-in-the-internet-age/ch6-let-food-be-thy-medicine

Kinney, K. (2015, October 8). *SIBO diet: What is it and can it treat the condition?* Chris Kresser. https://chriskresser.com/why-diet-alone-is-not-enough-to-treat-sibo/

Knezevic, J., Starchl, C., Tmava Berisha, A., & Amrein, K. (2020). Thyroid-gut-axis: How does the microbiota influence thyroid function? *Nutrients, 12*(6), 1769. https://doi.org/10.3390/nu12061769

Kotifani, A. (2022, November 10). *What is inflammation? The good and the bad*. Blue Zones. https://www.bluezones.com/2022/11/what-is-inflammation-the-good-and-the-bad/

Krans, B. (2019, August 16). *America's deadly sugar addiction has reached epidemic levels*. Healthline. https://www.healthline.com/health/sugar/americas-deadly-sugar-addiction

Kresser, C. (2017, November 15). *The gut-hormone connection: How gut microbes influence estrogen levels*. Kresser Institute. https://kresserinstitute.com/gut-hormone-connection-gut-microbes-influence-estrogen-levels/

Lacasse, S. (2012, March 1). *Quick and easy quinoa orange salad*. The Healthy Foodie. https://thehealthyfoodie.com/quick-and-easy-quinoa-orange-salad/

Lachtrupp, E. (2022, September 28). *Anti-inflammatory meal plan for beginners*. Eating Well. https://www.eatingwell.com/article/7894310/anti-inflammatory-meal-plan-for-beginners/

LaRoche, L. (2011, September 20). *Food can be a curse – and a cure.* Wicked Local. https://www.wickedlocal.com/story/bulletin-tab/2011/09/20/loretta-laroche-food-can-be/65327433007/

Lawler, M. (2020, June 29). *What is an anti-inflammatory diet? Benefits, food list, and tips.* Everyday Health. https://www.everydayhealth.com/diet-nutrition/diet/anti-inflammatory-diet-benefits-food-list-tips/

Lee, C. J., Sears, C. L., & Maruthur, N. (2019). Gut microbiome and its role in obesity and insulin resistance. *Annals of the New York Academy of Sciences, 1461*(1), 37–52. https://doi.org/10.1111/nyas.14107

Leonard, J. (2018, May 28). *10 research-backed ways to improve gut health.* Medical News Today. https://www.medicalnewstoday.com/articles/325293

Levy, J. (2020, November). *Vegan lentil soup.* Eating Well. https://www.eatingwell.com/recipe/7873236/vegan-lentil-soup/

Lewis, K. M. (2020, September 16). *Helping patients with diabetes manage stress.* National Institute of Diabetes and Digestive and Kidney Diseases. https://www.niddk.nih.gov/health-information/professionals/diabetes-discoveries-practice/helping-patients-with-diabetes-manage-stress#:~:text=The%20experience%20of%20stress%20might

Lifestyle changes for improved health - How to make healthy lifestyle changes. (n.d.). Delight Medical. https://www.delightmedical.com/wellness-guide/lifestyle-changes-for-improved-health

Lipman, F. (2022, July 26). *Overcoming sugar addiction.* Goop. https://goop.com/wellness/health/overcoming-sugar-addiction/

Lobionda, S., Sittipo, P., Kwon, H. Y., & Lee, Y. K. (2019). The role of gut microbiota in intestinal inflammation with respect to diet and extrinsic stressors. *Microorganisms*, *7*(8), 271. https://doi.org/10.3390/microorganisms7080271

Luciano, M. (2018, June 4). *6 vital organs to detox for optimum health*. Sun Warrior. https://sunwarrior.com/a/s/blogs/health-hub/6-vital-organs-to-detox-for-optimum-health

Mandal, A. (2009, December 3). *History of diabetes*. News-Medical. https://www.news-medical.net/amp/health/History-of-Diabetes.aspx

Mayo Clinic Staff. (2022a). *Small intestinal bacterial overgrowth (SIBO) - Symptoms and causes*. Mayo Clinic. https://www.mayoclinic.org/diseases-conditions/small-intestinal-bacterial-overgrowth/symptoms-causes/syc-20370168#:~:text=Small%20intestinal%20bacterial%20overgrowth%20(SIBO)%20can%20cause%20escalating%20problems%2C

Mayo Clinic Staff. (2022b, November 2). *Low-glycemic index diet: What's behind the claims?* Mayo Clinic. https://www.mayoclinic.org/healthy-lifestyle/nutrition-and-healthy-eating/in-depth/low-glycemic-index-diet/art-20048478#:~:text=Low%20GI%20%3A%20Green%20vegetables%2C%20most

Mayo Clinic Staff. (2020a, August 25). *Paleo diet: Eat like a cave man and lose weight?* Mayo Clinic. https://www.mayoclinic.org/healthy-lifestyle/nutrition-and-healthy-eating/in-depth/paleo-diet/art-20111182

Mayo Clinic Staff. (2020b, September 29). *Can triglycerides affect my heart health?* Mayo Clinic. https://www.mayoclinic.org/diseases-conditions/high-blood-cholesterol/in-depth/triglycerides/art-20048186

Mohammadi, D. (2014, December 5). *You can't detox your body. It's a myth. So how do you get healthy?* The Guardian. https://amp.theguardian.com/lifeandstyle/2014/dec/05/detox-myth-health-diet-science-ignorance

Moore, W. (2021, September 6). *Could insulin-resistance diet lower your diabetes risk?* Web MD. https://www.webmd.com/diabetes/diabetes-insulin-resistance-diet#:~:text=You%20don

National Heart, Lung, and Blood Institute. (2019). *Calculate your BMI - Standard BMI calculator.* NHLBI. https://www.nhlbi.nih.gov/health/educational/lose_wt/BMI/bmicalc.htm

National Institute of Diabetes and Digestive and Kidney Diseases. (2018, November 30). *Changing your habits for better health.* NIDDK. https://www.niddk.nih.gov/health-information/diet-nutrition/changing-habits-better-health

Naturopathic & holistic gut health. (n.d.). Dr. Lana Wellness. https://www.drlanawellness.com/conditions/gut-health

New Harbinger Publications. (2013, November 6). *7 ways to detox to reverse prediabetes.* HuffPost. https://www.huffpost.com/entry/preventing-prediabetes_b_4184272/amp

Newman, T. (2020, November 16). *Diabetes: Dispelling 11 common myths.* Medical News Today. https://www.medicalnewstoday.com/articles/medical-myths-all-about-diabetes

NHS. (2019). *Going for regular check-ups.* NHS. https://www.nhs.uk/conditions/type-2-diabetes/going-regular-check-ups/

NIDDK. (2017, November). *Eating, diet, & nutrition for irritable bowel syndrome.* National Institute of Diabetes and Digestive and Kidney Diseases. https://www.niddk.nih.gov/health-information/digestive-diseases/irritable-bowel-syndrome/eating-diet-nutrition#:~:text=with%20a%20dietitian.-

NIDDK. (2019, March 6). *Risk factors for type 2 diabetes.* National Institute of Diabetes and Digestive and Kidney Diseases. https://www.niddk.nih.gov/health-information/diabetes/overview/risk-factors-type-2-diabetes

NIH. (2013, December). *Control the ABCs of diabetes.* National Heart, Lung, and Blood Institute. https://www.nhlbi.nih.gov/health/educational/healthdisp/pdf/tipsheets/Control-the-ABCs-of-Diabetes.pdf

Norris, T. (2018, September 29). *Probiotics and digestive health: Benefits, risks, and more.* Healthline. https://www.healthline.com/health/probiotics-and-digestive-health

NorthShore University Health System. (2019, April 19). *Diet do's and don'ts with IBS.* North Shore. https://www.northshore.org/healthy-you/diet-dos-and-donts-with-ibs/

Northwestern Medicine. (n.d.). *7 reasons to listen to your gut.* Northwestern Medicine. https://www.nm.org/healthbeat/healthy-tips/7-reasons-to-listen-to-your-gut

Nunez, K. (2022, December 21). *8 sneaky signs you're walking around with poor gut health.* Real Simple. https://www.realsimple.com/signs-of-poor-gut-health-6951072

O'Connor, A. (2022, September 20). The best foods to feed your gut microbiome. *Washington Post.* https://www.washingtonpost.com/wellness/2022/09/20/gut-health-microbiome-best-foods/

Osborn, C. O. (2020, January 7). *Low histamine diet.* Healthline. https://www.healthline.com/health/low-histamine-diet

Paddock, C. (2009, January 5). *Debunking the detox myth.* Www.medicalnewstoday.com. https://www.medicalnewstoday.com/articles/134385#1

Pancreatic Cancer Action Network. (n.d.). *Diabetes and pancreatic cancer.* Pancreatic Cancer Action Network. https://pancan.org/facing-pancreatic-cancer/living-with-pancreatic-cancer/diet-and-nutrition/diabetes-and-pancreatic-cancer/

Pancreatic conditions - Pancreas disease. (n.d.). UCLA Health. https://www.uclahealth.org/medical-services/pancreas-disease/pancreatic-conditions

Pasqui, F., Poli, C., Magrino, C., & Festi, D. (2016). *Dietary management in IBS patients.* IntechOpen. https://www.intechopen.com/chapters/53002

Pathak, N. (2019). *Slideshow: How your gut health affects your whole body.* Web MD. https://www.webmd.com/digestive-disorders/ss/slideshow-how-gut-health-affects-whole-body

Patino, E. (2020, June 10). *Signs of an unhealthy gut and what you can do about it.* Everyday Health. https://www.everydayhealth.com/digestive-health/signs-of-unhealthy-gut-and-how-to-fix-it/

Peach State Health Plan. (2018, November 5). *Know your diabetes ABCs.* Pshpgeorgia. https://www.pshpgeorgia.com/newsroom/know-your-diabetes-abcs.html

Pelletier, S. (2015, January 2). *Hormone deficiency can drive sugar cravings.* Rock Creek Wellness. https://rockcreekwellness.com/hormone-deficiency-can-drive-sugar-cravings/amp/

Peters, A. (2012). Does sugar addiction really cause obesity? *Frontiers in Neuroenergetics, 3.* https://doi.org/10.3389/fnene.2011.00011

Petre, A. (2019, January 22). *The microbiome diet review: Food lists, benefits, and meal plan.* Healthline. https://www.healthline.com/nutrition/microbiome-diet

Piemonte, L. (2019, September 13). *Anti-inflammatory foods essential for diabetes.* Diabetes Voice. https://diabetesvoice.org/en/caring-for-diabetes/anti-inflammatory-foods-essential-for-diabetes/

Porter, E. (2012, January 26). *History of diabetes.* Healthline. https://www.healthline.com/health/history-type-1-diabetes

Prediabetes. (n.d.). Cleveland Clinic. https://my.clevelandclinic.org/health/diseases/21498-prediabetes

Reichelt, A. (2017, February 22). *Fact or fiction – is sugar addictive?* The Conversation. https://theconversation.com/amp/fact-or-fiction-is-sugar-addictive-73340

Richmond Natural Medicine. (n.d.). *Gastrointestinal health.* Richmond Natural Med. Retrieved January 18, 2023, from https://richmondnaturalmed.com/gastrointestinal-health-2/

Robertson, R. (2016, November 18). *10 ways to improve your gut bacteria, based on science.* Healthline. https://www.healthline.com/nutrition/improve-gut-bacteria

Robertson, R. (2020, August 20). *The gut-brain connection: How it works and the role of nutrition.* Healthline. https://www.healthline.com/nutrition/gut-brain-connection

Rocky Mountain Analytical. (2018, November 14). *The four R's of gut healing.* RM Lab. https://rmalab.com/the-four-rs-of-gut-healing/#:~:text=There%20are%20many%20factors%20that

Rocky Mountain Analytical. (n.d.). *Good vs. bad inflammation.* RM Lab. https://rmalab.com/good-vs-bad-inflammation/

Ruscio, M. (2020, October 10). *SIBO diets: Your guide to choosing the right one.* Drruscio.com. https://drruscio.com/sibo-diet/

Ruscio, M. (2022a, January 24). *What are the signs you need probiotics? How to help your gut.* Dr Ruscio. https://drruscio.com/what-are-the-signs-you-need-probiotics/

Ruscio, M. (2022b, April 23). *SIBO and your diet: What foods should be avoided with SIBO*. Dr Ruscio. https://drruscio.com/what-foods-should-be-avoided-with-sibo/

Sachdev, A. H., & Pimentel, M. (2013). Gastrointestinal bacterial overgrowth: pathogenesis and clinical significance. *Therapeutic advances in chronic disease*, *4*(5), 223–231. https://doi.org/10.1177/2040622313496126

Saha, S. (2020, November 18). *Manage diabetes: 7 amazing detox water recipes you can try*. NDTV. https://food.ndtv.com/diabetes/7-detox-water-recipes-for-diabetes-2326838/amp/1

Saleh, N. (2017). *12 benefits of detoxing the body*. Evoke Acupuncture. https://evokeacupuncture.com/12-benefits-of-detoxing-the-body/amp/

Schaefer, A., & Yasin, K. (2020, April 29). *Experts agree: Sugar might be as addictive as cocaine*. Healthline. https://www.healthline.com/health/food-nutrition/experts-is-sugar-addictive-drug

Scheithauer, T. P. M., Rampanelli, E., Nieuwdorp, M., Vallance, B. A., Verchere, C. B., van Raalte, D. H., & Herrema, H. (2020). Gut microbiota as a trigger for metabolic inflammation in obesity and type 2 diabetes. *Frontiers in Immunology*, *11*. https://doi.org/10.3389/fimmu.2020.571731

Scherneck, S. (2023, January 3). Special issue: Diabetes mellitus (DM) - Endocrine and metabolic disorders. *International Journal of Molecular Sciences*. https://www.mdpi.com/journal/ijms/special_issues/Diabetes_Metabolic

Scott, L. A. (n.d.). *Gut health and hormones*. Leigh Ann Scott MD, Las Colinas, Irving TX. Retrieved January 14, 2023, from https://www.leighannscottmd.com/additional-testing/gut-health-and-hormones/#:~:text=There%20is%20a%20link%20between

Searor, S. (2022, March 31). *The MIND, DASH, and Mediterranean diets -- What's the difference?* Your Memore. https://yourmemore.com/blogs/news/the-mind-dash-and-mediterranean-diets-what-s-the-difference#:~:text=The%20DASH%20eating%20plan%20is

Seidenberg, C. (2018, January 30). *Why we crave sugar, and how to beat the habit.* Washington Post. https://www.washingtonpost.com/lifestyle/wellness/explaining-the-siren-song-of-sugar-and-how-to-beat-the-habit/2018/01/26/8a9557f8-f7ae-11e7-a9e3-ab18ce41436a_story.html

Selah Medi Spa. (n.d.). *5 benefits of detoxing.* Selah Medispa https://www.selahmedispa.com/blog/5-benefits-of-detoxing

Sepel, J. (2017, September 16). *Gut-healing dinner recipe.* Mind Body Green. https://www.mindbodygreen.com/articles/gut-healing-dinner-recipe

Sheehan, K. (2018, December 6). *Craving for sugar in the morning.* SF Gate. https://healthyeating.sfgate.com/craving-sugar-morning-8579.html

Shen, J., Obin, M. S., & Zhao, L. (2013). The gut microbiota, obesity and insulin resistance. *Molecular Aspects of Medicine, 34*(1), 39–58. https://doi.org/10.1016/j.mam.2012.11.001

Shoelson, S. E., Lee, J., & Goldfine, A. B. (2006). Inflammation and insulin resistance. *Journal of Clinical Investigation, 116*(7), 1793–1801. https://doi.org/10.1172/jci29069

Shrivastava, S., Shrivastava, P., & Ramasamy, J. (2013). Role of self-care in management of diabetes mellitus. *Journal of Diabetes & Metabolic Disorders, 12*(1), 14. https://doi.org/10.1186/2251-6581-12-14

Snyder, W. (2015, February 10). *The good, the bad and the ugly of inflammation.* Vanderbilt Medicine. https://medschool.vanderbilt.edu/vanderbilt-medicine/the-good-the-bad-and-the-ugly-of-inflammation/#:~:text=When%20it

Solan, M. (2018, May 24). *Move more every day to combat a sedentary lifestyle.* Harvard Health Blog. https://www.health.harvard.edu/blog/move-more-every-day-to-combat-a-sedentary-lifestyle-2018052413913

Spritzler, F. (2018). *Anti-inflammatory diet 101: How to reduce inflammation naturally.* Healthline. https://www.healthline.com/nutrition/anti-inflammatory-diet-101

St. Kilda Osteopathy. (2020, February 13). *Being sedentary and being active.* St Kilda Osteopathy. https://www.stkildaosteopathy.com.au/blog/sedentary-vs-active-lifestyle/

Steiner, G. (1972). Diabetes mellitus: current concepts of the hormonal and metabolic defects. *Canadian Medical Association Journal, 107*(6), 539 passim. https://www.ncbi.nlm.nih.gov/pmc/articles/PMC1940914/

Stockwell, A. (2018, March 5). *Lentil and chicken soup with sweet potatoes and escarole.* Epicurious. https://www.epicurious.com/recipes/food/views/lentil-and-chicken-soup-with-sweet-potatoes-and-escarole

Strong, R., & Proctor, K. (2021, July 23). *Insulin resistance: Diet tips and 7-day meal plan.* Insider. https://www.insider.com/guides/health/diet-nutrition/insulin-resistance-diet?amp

Study Finds. (2022, October 20). *Diabetes, arthritis, and multiple sclerosis trace their roots back to the Black Death.* Study Finds. https://studyfinds.org/autoimmune-disease-black-death/

Takase, M. (2007). Complications of chronic inflammation. *Pancreas - Pathological Practice and Research,* 164–170. https://doi.org/10.1159/000100537

Taylor, K. (2019, April 20). *Homemade vegetarian chili.* Cookie and Kate. https://cookieandkate.com/vegetarian-chili-recipe/

Taylor, M. (2021, July 6). *Does sugar really cause inflammation?* Greatist. https://greatist.com/health/sugar-and-inflammation

Taylor, R. (2022, December 12). *What increases my risk of diabetes?* Web MD. https://www.webmd.com/diabetes/guide/risk-factors-for-diabetes

10 ways to strengthen your microbiome.(2022, August 4). Canadian Digestive Health Foundation. https://cdhf.ca/en/10-ways-to-strengthen-your-microbiome/

Thompson, S. (2016, May 23). *Sugar and chronic inflammation.* Sacred Vessel Acupuncture. https://www.sacredvesselacupuncture.com/educatethrive/understanding-the-important-role-sugar-plays-in-causing-and-pertetuating-chronic-inflammatory-conditions-day-4-menu-plan

Thursby, E., & Juge, N. (2017). Introduction to the human gut microbiota. *Biochemical Journal, 474*(11), 1823–1836. https://doi.org/10.1042/bcj20160510

Travers, C. (2022, November 27). *4 sneaky reasons you crave sugar + what to eat instead.* Mind Body Green. https://www.mindbodygreen.com/articles/craving-sugar

Types of diabetes. (2022b). Diabetes UK. https://www.diabetes.org.uk/diabetes-the-basics/types-of-diabetes

USC Department of Nursing. (2018, January 9). *What does self-care mean for diabetic patients?* Nursing. https://nursing.usc.edu/blog/self-care-with-diabetes/

Valdes, A. M., Walter, J., Segal, E., & Spector, T. D. (2018). Role of the gut microbiota in nutrition and health. *BMJ, 361*(361), k2179. https://doi.org/10.1136/bmj.k2179

Van De Walle, G. (2019, March 11). *Full body detox: 9 ways to rejuvenate your body.* Healthline. https://www.healthline.com/nutrition/how-to-detox-your-body

Varney, J. (2016, November 8). *Dietary fibre series - insoluble fibre.* Monash FODMAP. https://www.monashfodmap.com/blog/dietary-fibre-series-insoluble-fibre/

Veloso, H. (n.d.). *FODMAP diet: What you need to know.* Www.hopkinsmedicine.org. Retrieved January 19, 2023, from https://www.hopkinsmedicine.org/health/wellness-and-prevention/fodmap-diet-what-you-need-to-know

Waghorn, M. (2022, October 19). *Black Death may have fuelled rise in diabetes and arthritis, study says.* The Independent. https://www.independent.co.uk/independentpremium/world/diabetes-arthritis-plague-study-b2207125.html

Walker, C. (2015). *The effects of an American diet on health.* UAB. https://www.uab.edu/inquiro/issues/past-issues/volume-9/the-effects-of-an-american-diet-on-health

Wang, J., Chen, W.-D., & Wang, Y.-D. (2020). The relationship between gut microbiota and inflammatory diseases: The role of macrophages. *Frontiers in Microbiology, 11.* https://doi.org/10.3389/fmicb.2020.01065

Wang, X., Zhang, P., & Zhang, X. (2021). Probiotics regulate gut microbiota: An effective method to improve immunity. *Molecules, 26*(19), 6076. https://doi.org/10.3390/molecules26196076

Ward, E. (2022, June 29). *How to keep your gut microbiome healthy.* Web MD. https://blogs.webmd.com/heart-health/20220629/keep-your-gut-microbiome-healthy

Washington, R. (2016, January 4). *This 2-minute detox drink helps you burn fat, fight diabetes and lower blood pressure.* My Houston Majic. https://myhoustonmajic.com/3169031/this-2-minute-detox-drink-helps-you-burn-fat-fight-diabetes-and-lower-blood-pressure/amp/

Webster, K. (2017, October). *Stuffed sweet potato with hummus dressing.* Eating Well. https://www.eatingwell.com/recipe/260717/stuffed-sweet-potato-with-hummus-dressing/

Wedro, B. (2022, August 8). *SIBO (gut bacteria problem) symptoms, causes, antibiotic, probiotic treatment.* Medicine Net. https://www.medicinenet.com/small_intestinal_bacterial_over growth_sibo/article.htm

Wieërs, G., Belkhir, L., Enaud, R., Leclercq, S., Philippart de Foy, J.-M., Dequenne, I., de Timary, P., & Cani, P. D. (2020). How probiotics affect the microbiota. *Frontiers in Cellular and Infection Microbiology, 9*(454). https://doi.org/10.3389/fcimb.2019.00454

Wilson, C. (2022, October 16). *Food can be the curse or the cure.* InkFreeNews.com. https://www.inkfreenews.com/2022/10/16/food-can-be-the-curse-or-the-cure/

Wiss, D. A., Avena, N., & Rada, P. (2018). Sugar addiction: From evolution to revolution. *Frontiers in Psychiatry, 9.* https://doi.org/10.3389/fpsyt.2018.00545

Wong, C. (2022, April 18). *What should you eat for an anti-inflammatory diet?* Verywell Health. https://www.verywellhealth.com/anti-inflammatory-diet-88752

Woodle, J. M. (n.d.). *The 4 R's: How to heal and restore your gut naturally.* Www.assuaged.com. Retrieved January 16, 2023, from https://www.assuaged.com/news/the-4-rs-how-to-heal-and-restore-your-gut-naturally

Woodyard, A. (2021, December 17). *Dash diet vs Mediterranean diet 2022.* Meal Plan Pros. https://mealplanpros.com/dash-diet-vs-mediterranean-diet/

World Diabetes Foundation. (n.d.). *Understanding diabetes & self care guideline*. World Diabetes Foundation. Retrieved January 24, 2023, from https://www.worlddiabetesfoundation.org/sites/default/files/ Understanding%20diabetes%20&%20Self%20care%20guidelin e_WDF03-060.pdf

Wu, H., & Ballantyne, C. M. (2020). Metabolic inflammation and insulin resistance in obesity. *Circulation Research*, *126*(11), 1549– 1564. https://doi.org/10.1161/circresaha.119.315896

Zaremba, K. (2021). *The 4Rs: How to heal your gut naturally*. Full Script. https://fullscript.com/blog/natural-gut-healing/amp

Image References

Barbhuiya, T. (2021). White digital device beside white pen photo. https://unsplash.com/photos/ZJaK9jQXeDA

Bluewater Sweden. (2020). Person in blue denim jacket holding stainless steel bottle photo. https://unsplash.com/photos/4Kd3svPFuEI

CA Creative. (2018). Grilled fish, cooked vegetables, and fork on plate photo. https://unsplash.com/photos/bpPTlXWTOvg

Đurić, Z. (2020). Fruits and vegetables in clear glass jar photo. https://unsplash.com/photos/U4QkDQW84sg

Feinkost, K. (2020). Cooked food on black frying pan photo. In *Unsplash*. https://unsplash.com/photos/B7_QFoTCunE

Ghosh, R. (2020). Free india image. https://unsplash.com/photos/NPrWYa69Mz0

Hansel, L. (2019). Tray of food on white surface photo. https://unsplash.com/photos/K47107aP8UU

Horn, M. W. (2017). Clear jar filled with lemonade juice photo. https://unsplash.com/photos/lo_udD1o_lk

Калегин, M. (2016). Woman sleeping on trailer photo. https://unsplash.com/photos/ffustAcaX0E

Kudriavtseva, O. (2020). Strawberries in white ceramic bowl photo. https://unsplash.com/photos/s8J1DlRroo0

Lark, B. (2017). Poached egg with vegetables and tomatoes on blue plate photo. https://unsplash.com/photos/jUPOXXRNdcA

Lauch, L. (2019). Two fried eggs photo. https://unsplash.com/photos/osPCHdpXKxk

Little plant. (2021). Clear glass jars with candies photo. I https://unsplash.com/photos/TZw891-oMio

Macey, D. (2018). Yellow corn on glass bowl photo. https://unsplash.com/photos/h83Rm3njjcg

Olinger, H. (2018). Woman sitting in front of black table writing on white book near window photo. https://unsplash.com/photos/NXiIVnzBwZ8

Plenio, J. (2021). Woman in white jacket and black pants walking on road during daytime photo. https://unsplash.com/photos/pxEroa7lYx8

Rasyid, F. (2018). Pile of grocery items photo. https://unsplash.com/photos/ezeC8-clZSs

Shes, V. (2019). Cooked food photo. https://unsplash.com/photos/wSh0Exrb62g

Skydsgaard, M. (2021). Person wearing white and yellow sneakers photo. https://unsplash.com/photos/_A7WLos9RfU

Sorge, R. (2016). Clear glass cruet bottle photo. https://unsplash.com/photos/uOBApnN_K7w

Made in the USA
Las Vegas, NV
28 May 2024